Life Part Two:

Life Part Two:

Living a Healthy and Happier Retirement

A Guide to Assist in Planning and Transitioning

Throughout Retirement

Mark A. Brimer Ph.D.

ISBN 9781070543475

To Leslee: my wife and best friend

Table of Contents

Introduction

For nearly 40 years, as a healthcare professional, I have had the opportunity to work with patients who are approaching the age of retirement or have already retired. Throughout the years, I noticed that some people were very prepared to retire while others struggled with retirement preparation and retirement itself. I began examine why some people seemed to adjust well to retirement while others seemingly struggled. The goal of under-taking this clinical examination was to determine if there are obvious reasons why retirement is "great for some" and "not so great for others."

In the process of examining retirement I observed a pattern that emerged for those people who were the "most satisfied with retirement." The most satisfied seemed to engage in three (3) specific activities on a regular basis. These three activities led to the development of the HAP Retirement Model. The HAP Model is designed as common sense tool to help you, or someone close to you, with ensuring retirement is as enjoyable as it can be. It is very important to point out, however, the HAP model has not been verified through any scientific or statistical testing but, rather, by clinical examination in the field through observation. At the most simple level, HAP is a tool that is designed to allow on-going self-examination and, therefore, better retirement planning.

The HAP Retirement Model has three letters that identify a cycle for increased life-satisfaction in retirement. Each letter of the model represents a position within retirement. For example the letter (H) stands for Health Examination, (A) Activity and Exercise, and (P) Planning for Change. HAP is an action orientated model that focuses upon the transitional processes that occur throughout retirement. The model has been created for use at any point of the retirement process to allow the user to focus upon preparing for and managing the changes encountered as we age.

For many, Life Part II begins with the decision to retire. Once the decision is made to retire the focus should change from the connection to career to the role as a non-worker. The decision to move from a worker to a non-worker becomes a transition. By utilizing the principles of HAP, retirement transition is accomplished in a meaningful manner that can be carried throughout life. Hopefully the HAP model will guide you in the personal identification of life elements to focus upon so your retirement will be as healthy, happy, safe, and enjoyable as possible.

Mark A. Brimer Ph.D.

Chapter 1

Where Retirement Should Begin

The first step to getting-off to a good start with retirement is determining what you want retirement to be. Retirement is no longer about sitting-around and watching television and relaxing as the years go by. A fulfilling retirement is best accomplished by having a plan. Without a plan many retirees report feeling unfilled and unsatisfied. Although an important part of the plan should include a review of your financial assets, the personal and emotional side of retirement is equally as important. The personal, emotional and physical side of retirement is what this book is about.

For many, the workplace was a reliable source of personal satisfaction, achievement, and accomplishment for the work that was completed. In your former employment position there may have been awards and recognition for a job well done. Rewards and recognition may have helped with making the decision of whether or not to get out of bed each-and-every-day a little easier. For some, work-days were filled with meetings and networking events which provided opportunities to interact with colleagues, socialize, and make friends. Some of the work-day interactions also offered outside social opportunities that lasted for many years.

Once you leave the workplace your retirement plan needs to include how to fill the void that was occupied by 40 hours or more a week for many years. This chapter identifies ways to help you find meaning as you enter and move through the months and years of a happy and healthy retirement.

Find a Meaning and Purpose for the 2nd Part of Your Life.

Having a sense of meaning can be a key factor in experiencing happiness (1). The concept of happiness changes with aging. In our younger years we typically associated the feeling of happiness with excitement. With aging, however, we often associate happiness with peace (2). One possible reason why there is a shift in the feelings of happiness is because there may be a change in focus from the future to the present with aging (3).

Purpose and meaning are encouraged by 4 main life experiences(4):

Physical and mental well-being

Belonging and recognition

Personally treasured activities

Spiritual closeness and connectedness

Physical and mental well-being means caring for your body and mind. This can be accomplished by lowering the stress levels that may have predominated work-life. The concept of **belonging and recognition** refers to feeling valued and validated.

Personally treasured activities are the things that you enjoy and that make you feel good. These activities may include hobbies and spending time with special friends and family. **Spiritual closeness and connectedness** is the feeling that all living things in the world are connected to one-another.

Plan by Visualizing Your Future

For some, one of the most difficult aspects of retirement is planning for the future. Historically, shorter activities such as planning for a vacation seldom create problems for us; most can handle that type of planning activity. But planning for 20-30 years down the road in retirement can be difficult to envision.   To help visualize your future in retirement try **writing down** answers the following questions:

> How will your daily routine change? What do you see yourself doing at the beginning of the day?

> How will you spend your time?

> Is it possible you will return to work?

> Who do you see spending most of your time with?

> Where do you plan to live? Is the location you plan to live your best choice?

> Will you take any steps to improve your health?

The idea behind answering these questions is that it brings-to-life the reality of how retirement is likely to develop. One of your goals should be to spend your time doing the activities that most interest you. Answering these questions in a meaningful way will also assist in the identification of the financial resources needed to attain your goals.

Another important activity to do with the answers to these questions is to share them with those closest to you. For example, if you are married your spouse should also answer the questions. His or her answers may reflect an entirely different meaning, purpose, or set of objectives for retirement than you have. If so, the differences in desires and plans should be discussed and a compromise reached so each of you has an opportunity to experience the best of retirement.

Health and Retirement Satisfaction: They Go Hand-in-Hand

According to a study conducted by Merrill Lynch in partnership with Age Wave, 81% of retirees believe health is the most important ingredient for happy retirement. Baby boomers are 2 ½ times more likely to say they are proactive about their health and to view their doctors as partners who work with them to optimize their health (5).

Five Strategies listed in the Merrill Lynch – Age Wave report for healthier aging included:

1. Exercise – Seniors who begin exercising in their 60's or 70's are 3 times more likely to age healthfully compared to seniors who don't.

2. Healthier Diet – Reduces the risk of strokes, diabetes, and cancer.

3. A Healthy Weight – Those aged 45-64 who exercise and maintain a proper diet, reduce the risk of heart disease by 35%.

4. Socialization – Low levels of social interaction can be just as unhealthy as smoking, obesity, or insufficient levels of exercise.

5. Avoid Poor Habits – These include smoking, excessive alcohol drinking, and stress.

Part of planning for a healthy and happier retirement means taking an active role in making change. Although change can be difficult it is always recommended to proceed slowly and one day at a time. To assist in the change processes, it may be beneficial to visualize a strong emotional reason for the change. For example, "I need to make this change soon otherwise it may impact my ability to travel and spend quality time with my family." Creating an emotional link for the change may provide you a stronger reason to embrace and proceed with change.

A Bump-in-the-Road Requires a Positive Outlook

With aging we often encounter issues that can de-rail even the best retirement plans. Some of the most likely retirement issues encountered will be those that interrupt health. How we respond to the issues encountered is vital to how we move forward and continue to experience a rewarding retirement. One study demonstrated that seniors with a positive attitude toward themselves are 44% more likely to fully recover from an experience with physical disability than someone with a negative outlook (6). Three additional suggestions include:

1. Examine the Problem/Situation. Is the bump-in-the-road really that significant or will the problem just necessitate more effort on your part? As quickly as possible, try to come to terms with the problem and begin planning next steps. Commit yourself to taking ownership and, if necessary, ask for advice and assistance. You may find there are others willing to offer assistance. Consider taking their help.

2. Review How Far You Have Come. Instead of viewing the problem at hand as a retirement failure, take a moment and recognize how far you have come. In your younger years, you had to over-come obstacles and problems in order to reach the age of retirement. Make it a mission to fully address the problem and identify possible solutions.

5

3. Remain Goal Focused. You can be productive and useful at any age as long as you are planning for tomorrow. Periodically you may need to adjust your goals to reach a desired target. As a reminder, a set-back is little or nothing in the big scheme of things if you really want something and are willing to work to reach your goals.

Establish a Schedule and Stick to It. Some of the happiest and most fulfilled people in retirement are those that develop a retirement schedule and stick to it. You may have spent 30 to 40 years following a routine of working 8 AM to 5 PM and the thought of developing a "new" routine may have no appeal what-so-ever. Retirement is a major life-change but, with an established schedule you can avoid feeling restless and bored. The feelings of restlessness and boredom result from moving away from a career to a life provided with activities only when you initiate them. For many, having no routine can be far more mentally, physically, and emotionally draining than creating and following a new routine. Here are some tips for building a new post-retirement routine:

1.   Create a Daily To-Do List – Write down the things you want to accomplish in the day. Identifying what you want to accomplish allows you to get more out of the day rather than just going along performing random tasks. Additionally, as you cross-off the tasks on the list, you're more likely to experience a sense of accomplishment.

2.   Build Good Activity Habits – Once a decision has been made regarding desired daily activities, you're more likely to experience happiness and increased productivity. For example, long periods of inactivity such as unlimited time in front of the television are not good for your health. Some retirees begin the day seated in front of the television and remain seated there for the entire day. The more inactive retirement becomes the more rapidly your health is likely to deteriorate.

3. Practice Good Sleep Habits – Sleep is very important to our health. The short term lack of sleep will affect mood, judgement, and the ability to retain information. Some studies have shown a chronic loss of sleep may lead to increased risk of diabetes, cardiovascular disease, and obesity. The most common recommended time period for sleep is no less than 7 hours.

In the book "The Harvard Medical School Guide to a Good Night's Sleep" co-authors Dr.'s Lawrence Epstein and Mardron Steven have two recommendations for healthy sleep(7):

1. Get no less than 7 hours of sleep
2. As much as possible, get your sleep during the same time frame each day.

Having an active routine is also another important aspect of helping to get a good night's sleep. The more mentally and physically active you are throughout the day, and by avoiding napping, the more likely you are to rest comfortably at night.

Visit the Best Places to Retire

Each year rankings are presented that identify the best places to live when you retire. If you think your retirement should include relocation from your current residence, you'll need to evaluate the suitability of each potential location. Here are 15 questions to consider with each location visited:

1. Will the climate for the location work for you – year around?

2. What type of house would you like to live in? Some of the most popular options include: a condo, town-home, or an apartment.

3. Do you want a yard? Does your pet need a location to walk?

4. Is the community safe and secure? Is this a gated community?

5. Is there a location close by, that is lighted and safe so you can park your car?

6. Is there public transportation in-case you are unable to drive?

7. Will state or local taxes be become a financial hard-ship on a fixed income?

8. If you decide to return to work, are there employment opportunities in your areas of interest?

9. Are you able to locate a physician to meet your medical needs? Does that physician accept new patients? Does the physician accept your health care insurance?

10. Do you have any special food requirements? Will the closest grocery store be able to meet your needs?

11. How accessible is the local hospital? Is there a pharmacy close by?

12. Can the community accommodate your hobbies? Is there a senior center close-by? Would you take part in the activities offered at a senior center?

13. Are there facilities close-by that meet your religious needs? Visit the facility.

14. If you anticipate caring for an ill or debilitated spouse, how accessible are support services?

15. Is there a fitness center close by? Will the equipment accommodate seniors? Is the cost for membership reasonable? Is the facility clean? Has it been in business for greater than one year? Does it look like it will remain in business?

When visiting potential retirement locations, imagine living there a minimum of 20 years (or longer). This is important because you may experience less mobility with advancing age. Although no community is perfect, you should have as a goal to reside in a community that offers every opportunity to remain in your home for as long as possible.

Retirement Travel Should Be a Top Priority

One of the first things many seniors want to do after beginning retirement is to travel. Planning and taking a trip immediately following retirement can be a great way to mentally and physically move away from the old job and ease into retirement. It is important to recognize, however, that travel should be built into your retirement plans not just initially but for the long term. The following are three suggestions to help in planning multiple vacations throughout your retirement:

1. Make a list of the places you would like to visit. For example, list the top ten places you'd like to visit and then begin determining which are likely to be the most enjoyable. Although visiting previous destinations may be enjoyable, travel at the retirement stage of life should be about seeing and doing something new. New experiences help make retirement develop into the "new phase of life."

2. Discuss proposed retirement plans with your spouse. Compare the list of locations you'd like to visit to the list developed by your spouse. Discuss how the lists could be combined to make the travel more enjoyable for both.

3. Most importantly, take time to plan the trip right. A well planned trip helps build anticipation. It also allows you to investigate potential sites to visit in each location before arriving. Effective planning is the key to a greater appreciation of what you are seeing and experiencing.

Take Time to Reflect But Don't Stay in Reflection

There are times when all of us want to reflect on our life. This includes talking with family and friends about your life's activities and accomplishments, reading old correspondence, and reviewing old pictures. Although this is normal activity to occasionally engage in, continually remaining in the "reflection mode of life" can eventually distance you from others. Discussing the past, or the difficulties associated with growing older can be a real turn-off to family and friends. Make it your goal to be positive about aging.

Being positive about aging is a process that can be developed over time. It can begin by spending time each day expressing gratitude for the many blessings that have come your way. Life may not have turned out exactly as planned but work to focus your attention upon the good things that have occurred and be appreciative for what you have.

Negative self-perceptions of aging have been shown to result in lower levels of preventative behavior, health, and longevity (8). On the other-hand, remaining positive with aging does have health benefits.

For example, the obesity epidemic among older adults is expected to continue unless there are efforts to help this age group. In one study the researchers investigated whether self-perceptions of aging, or the beliefs about oneself, could relate to new cases of obesity.

The study found that older persons with a more positive self-perception of aging were less likely to become obese over the next six years. In particular, a study participant with the most positive self-perception of aging score was 27% less likely to become obese than a same aged participant with an average self-perception score (9).

Developing the Social & Leisure Activity Side

One of the most important activities that you can do following retirement is to work on creating new friendships, increasing social relationships, and remaining active with leisure activities. Once retired many will keep in contact with friends from the former work setting but, over time, those contacts will also retire. Those friends may move on to other activities and cease to remain in contact.

There are many health benefits to creating and maintaining friendships and socialization with aging. Individuals with enhanced social relationships not only improve psychological well-being (e.g. by gaining a sense of belonging and lessening depression), but also physical health (e.g. by enhancing immune function and reducing heart attack risks) (10).

Participating in leisure activities in retirement that may be defined as; "preferred and enjoyable activities participated in during one's free time" (11). These activities represent a sense of freedom and provide intrinsic satisfaction (12). Leisure activities with others may provide social support, enrich meaning in life, assist recovery from stress, and help older adults adapt to potential restrictions caused by chronic health conditions(13), (14), (15), and (16).

Specific types of leisure activity may also be more beneficial than others. In one study five types of leisure activities for older adults were examined with regards to how participation affects health status. The leisure activities examined included; mental, social, physical, productive, and recreational activities. The researchers found that mental activities (e.g., writing, reading) were not only the most popular but also enhanced well-being the most (17).

In a study involving Swedish adults, researchers divided 15 leisure activities into six domains; culture-entertainment, productive-personal growth, outdoor-physical, recreation-expressive, friendship, and formal-group. The results determined that engaging in friendship-type leisure activities (e.g., visiting friends) resulted in the highest quality of life in older adults (18).

Another group of researchers conducted a review of literature on social and leisure activities and the well-being of older adults. The review concluded that informal social activity (e.g., going to clubs) benefited the well-being of older adults the most (19).

Pet Companionship

A pet can bring a lot of happiness into the life of a retired person and can also provide health benefits. Owning a pet can serve as an important source of social support, providing positive psychological benefits for their owners (19). An Australian survey found the expected potential benefits of dog ownership included; increased walking, happiness, companionship, decreased stress, and loneliness(21).

For adults 50 years and older one study demonstrated that pet ownership was associated with an improved cardiovascular disease survival in currently treated patients with high blood pressure (22), (23). When evaluating the potential benefit of owning a cat rather than a dog, other researchers determined owning a cat was significantly associated with a reduced hazard of dying from cardiovascular disease events, in particular a stroke (24). The protection a pet offers may not be simply from the physical activities but, due to the personality of the pet owners or stress-relieving effects of animal companionship (25).

Most Importantly – Have a Positive Aging Attitude

Successful aging depends greatly upon maintaining a positive attitude. A positive attitude about growing older can help you live longer and be more satisfied. Psychologist Becca Levy Ph.D., from Yale University conducted a study in the late 1990's and determined people with positive views on aging lived an average of 7.6 years longer than those with negative views (26).

Having a sense of purpose and happiness along with a positive attitude as an older adult helps to suppress negative thoughts and allows you to remain a productive member of society regardless of age or physical capabilities. When you encounter a challenging situation avoid negative self-talk. When the first thing you do is to think of is; "how bad it is" you have entered into the negative-thought pattern. Think first about the situation and less regarding how to react to it.

Remaining positive with aging is not about ignoring the reality of the situation. It is taking the opportunity to avoid thoughts of feeling hopeless or over-whelmed and shifts you towards an attitude of willingness to tackle life's challenges by looking for creative solutions to problems. Becoming successful shifting to a positive attitude as an older adult involves a life-long commitment to looking inside yourself and challenging negative thoughts. Once those thoughts are challenged you have the opportunity to make positive life changes.

The HAP Model for Retirement Planning & Transition

Life Part II is about getting the most out of life in every year of retirement. In order to do so, the *HAP Model for Retirement Planning and Transition* is designed to be a common sense guide to viewing retirement not as a destination but as a transition. As part of the transition, the model encourages you to think and plan for what is next in life.

To begin with, there is no publication that can guarantee retirement will always go the way we prepare. The basic idea of the HAP Model is to spend time using the 3 part transitional processes to help you visualize moving toward and through retirement. The goal is to encourage you to not spend time thinking about the career you are leaving behind but, on what you can do with the life that lies ahead.

The HAP Model begins with the assumption that people will likely live an additional 20-30 years beyond the traditional retirement age of 65 years. HAP is action orientated and a way of thinking about the steps we continually go through as we age. The basic idea presented by the HAP model is that each of the 3 components of the model will remain throughout the aging process and always be in a state of transition.

The 3 parts of the model are depicted as follows:

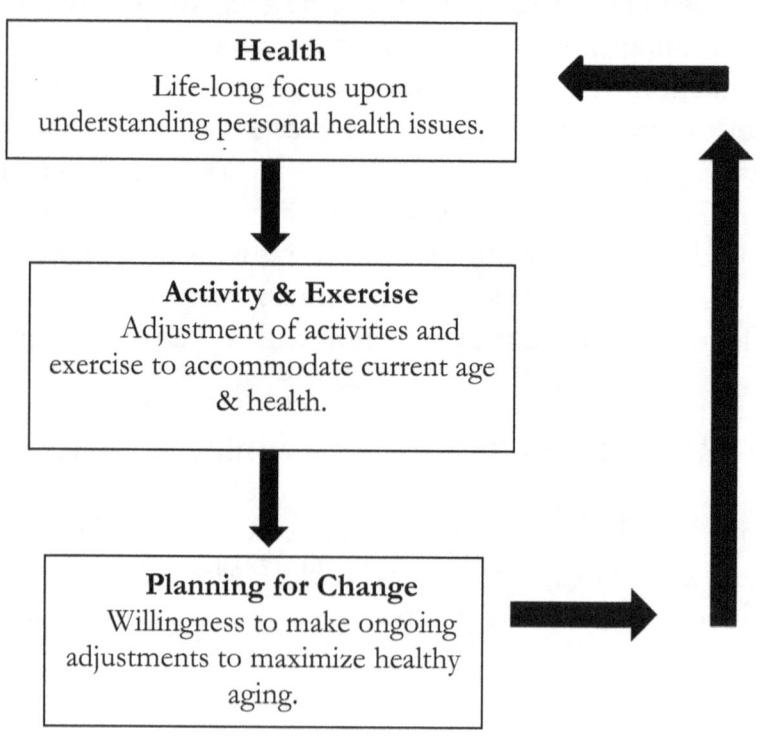

Health – "H" in the HAP model represents the on-going need to monitor your health. Once you have reached the age of retirement, your #1 responsibility is to monitor your health. Many of the changes you encounter with aging can be very manageable if you identify problems early and take action. The process of identifying problems, finding solutions, and taking action can be done by working hand-in-hand with your doctor. When you visit your doctor, simply ask the question; "How am I doing and what do I need to work-on?"

When your physician makes a new diagnosis and prescribes a treatment recommendation your role is to understand what is going-on with your aging body. With each year of aging, the human body changes in predictable and unpredictable ways. For example, a predicable change may involve making adjustments to prescribed medication to ensure good health is maintained. An unpredictable change may be the onset of a new diagnosis that requires treatment. The more you understand changing aspects of your health the more you can manage your retirement in healthy ways.

Activities & Exercise – The single most beneficial element for healthy aging is remaining active. Exercise is considered a key foundational component to healthy aging. This book covers the important aspects of healthy aging by explaining how regular exercise is essential for maintaining good health throughout retirement. Topics such as the benefits to increased physical activity, steps to take before initiating an exercise program, selection of the best exercises, and how to remain motivated to continue activity with aging are discussed. The importance of evaluating home safety is addressed and how small changes in the home can promote safety and healthy aging.

Planning for Change – Aging is a process that has up's-and-down's. The basis of the HAP Model is that physical activity will have to be refocused with aging and illness. For example, it is unlikely a 90 year old will be able to perform the same physical activities as a 65 year old. Because of the changes associated with aging the model recognizes that life as a retiree will always require transitional adjustment.

Chapter Summary

The common theme in this chapter is that retirement, in order to be the most enjoyable, cannot be a spectator sport. Simply by changing the way you think and the activities you participate in can have can have a favorable impact upon the quality of life. The top things to focus upon in retirement should include:

Seek to Find a Meaning and Purpose for the 2nd Part of Your Life

Plan Retirement by Visualizing Your Future

Work at Remaining Healthy

Expect Bumps-in-the-Road

Establish a Schedule and Stick to It

Consider Visiting the Best Places to Retire

Retirement Travel Should Be a Top Priority

Take Time to Reflect But Don't Stay in Reflection

Develop the Social & Leisure Side of Retirement

Consider Getting a Pet

Develop a Positive Aging Attitude

Making On-going Life Adjustments with the HAP Model

Chapter 2

The Benefits to Increased Physical Activity

One of the best things that you can do for yourself in retirement, regardless of age, is to exercise and remain physically active. Participation in regular exercise and physical activity is important to the physical and mental health of all age groups but is especially beneficial to older adults. Remaining physically active will allow you to continue participation in many of the activities you enjoy and provide for increased opportunities for independence as you age. As a matter of fact, when older people lose the ability to do things, it is not typically because they have aged. In many cases it is simply because they have become inactive.

This chapter focuses upon providing an understanding of the many benefits regular exercise has upon: cardiorespiratory fitness, preventing muscle loss, obesity, stroke, high blood pressure, diabetes, colon cancer, and musculoskeletal disorders. The chapter identifies the health benefits that can be obtained with exercise and increased physical activity.

One of the biggest challenges faced with the aging process is adopting a lifestyle that includes making choices of increased physical activity and exercise. Older adults have become aware that increased physical activity can improve health but there is often discussion regarding the type of benefits that can obtained with a regular physical activity and exercise program.

Physical activity and **exercise** are different terms that are often used to mean the same thing. **Physical activity** is defined as performing activities that help get the body moving. Physical activity includes: going for a walk, mowing the yard, cleaning out the garage, and taking the stairs rather than the elevator. **Exercise** is a form of physical activity but exercise is more structured so that activities are repetitive or concentrated on specific tasks. **Exercise** includes such activities as: weight training, resistive band training, endurance activities, and balance and flexibility training.

Physical inactivity is associated with deconditioning, weight gains, depression, and cardiovascular disease. It is important to note, however, that the negative effects of periods of prolonged inactivity can be reduced or potentially reversed by the adoption of exercise or increased physical activity. The positive benefits of exercise will be discussed by reviewing the impacts of the major systems associated with health.

Cardiovascular & Cardiorespiratory Diseases & Fitness

Those who are sedentary have nearly twice the risk of developing or dying from coronary heart disease. Studies show it is never too late to start being active. For example; regular physical activity and exercise does provide a beneficial effect on high density lipoprotein (HDL) cholesterol and can result in a reduction in systolic and diastolic blood pressure (1), (2).

Regular exercise contributes to longevity. Endurance exercise, including high-intensity training to improve cardiorespiratory fitness, promotes longevity and slows down aging (3). Additionally, endurance training in elderly populations was determined to be the most effective way to improve neuromuscular and cardiorespiratory functions (4).

Regular walking, such as on a golf course surface, can have a small training effect. Walking during a golf game is low risk for injury and a good form of health-enhancing physical activity (5). Golf may also lower total cholesterol and low-density lipoprotein cholesterol (LDL) levels (6).

Physical Activity and Stroke

A stroke occurs when the blood supply to part of your brain is interrupted or severely reduced, depriving the brain of oxygen. Some lifestyle risk factors associated with an increased risk for stroke include:

Being overweight or obese
Physical inactivity
Heavy or binge drinking
Use of illicit drugs such as cocaine and methamphetamines

There are two primary types of stroke; ischemic and hemorrhagic. Both types can be debilitating and significantly limit the quality of life for an older adult. Although approximately 80% of strokes are due to cerebral ischemia, physical activity may reduce the magnitude of injury from ischemic stroke so that there are fewer or less severe symptoms (7). The mechanisms for reduction of risk for stroke with increased physical activity may be due to either a decreased possibility of thrombus (clot) formation, or through reducing blood pressure levels.

The performance of aerobic or "cardio" exercise can reduce your risk of stroke in several ways. Similar to cardiovascular and cardiorespiratory disease, aerobic exercise can lower blood pressure, have positive effects on blood lipid levels, and improve overall blood vessel and heart health (8), (9). Aerobic exercise also assists with weight reduction and helps control diabetes and reduce stress.

Diabetes

It has been estimated that 33-50% of all new cases of Type 2 diabetes mellitus could be prevented by appropriate levels of physical activity (10). Type 2 diabetes or noninsulin-dependent diabetes, is a chronic condition that affects the way your body metabolizes sugar (glucose). With Type 2 diabetes the body either resists the effects of

19

insulin or doesn't produce sufficient insulin to maintain a normal glucose level. At present, there is no cure for Type 2 diabetes. It can however, be properly managed by eating well, exercising and maintaining a healthy weight. If diet and exercise aren't sufficient to manage blood sugar, medications or insulin therapy may be required.

A healthy lifestyle is essential to the prevention of Type 2 diabetes. Even if you have history of Type 2 diabetes in your family, adopting a healthy lifestyle and implementing a regular exercise program can help prevent the disease. If a diagnosis of Type 2 diabetes has already occurred, a healthy lifestyle choices and exercise can help prevent or slow the onset of many of the common complications. Four additional recommendations include:

1. Begin eating healthy foods. Select foods that are lower in fat and calories. Focus upon fruits, vegetables whole grains, and food that is high in fiber.

2. Increase physical activity. Start out slow and gradually progress to 30 minutes of physical activity a day. For example, take a brisk walk or ride a bike. If time availability is an issue, perform several 10-minute walks throughout the day.

3. Step on the scale. If overweight, losing body weight can reduce the risk of diabetes. To maintain a healthy weight, implement permanent changes to eating and make exercise a healthy habit.

4. For those with established type 2 diabetes, regular physical activity 3-4 times per week promotes muscle uptake of glucose and helps with diabetes control (11).

Declining Muscle Mass with Aging

The normal aging process is characterized by a decline in skeletal muscle mass which is responsible for a loss in strength (12). The loss of strength with aging may affect daily function, quality of life, independence, and significantly increases the risk of frailty and fracture. The most obvious reductions in strength often affect physical activities such as being able to rise from a chair or toilet seat, step over obstacles in the home or community, walk the required speed to safely to cross a street, or lift groceries into or out of a car. If the loss of strength continues without intervention, assistance may be required or some daily activities will need to be modified.

Individuals who have increased levels of physical activity with aging preserve muscle function better than those who don't. Older adults have the potential to increase muscle size and obtain strength gains with programs involving resistive training. Some of the important aspects concerning resistance training include:

1. To be effect, strength training needs to include the use of free weights, machine weights, body weight, or the use of elastic tubing or bands.

2. The performance of aerobic exercise, although very beneficial to increasing mobility and improving the cardiovascular system, has little effect on increasing muscle size or strength.

3. In order for a program of strength training to be effective it must be progressive in nature. For improving or maintaining function, it is important to target the major muscle groups of the body.

4. Endurance based exercise programs should focus upon the performance of higher repetitions through the full range of motion. If the goal is to increase power, heavier weights are recommended along with reduced repetitions.

The goal of performing a strength training program is to enhance or retain quality of life and independent function. Resistance training can enhance muscle function even with a frequency of performance of once or twice a week. If weights or machines are not available then home-made equipment such soda bottles or socks filled with sand or marbles may be used. The use of home-made equipment can be modified as strength and endurance continue to improve.

Obesity and Aging

Obesity is a disorder involving an excessive increase in body fat. If left untreated obesity increases the risk of health problems such as heart disease, joint pain, diabetes, kidney issues, high blood pressure, shortness of breath, and increased difficulty walking. Obesity can be particularly difficult to manage with increased age and lack of physical mobility (13).

In some instances genetic and or hormonal imbalances are responsible for increased body weight. When genetic or hormonal issues are not present, obesity will occur when more calories are consumed than are burned through exercise or normal daily activities. When calories are not burned, the body stores the excess number of calories as body fat. Dietary changes, increased physical activity, and behavior changes can help with weight loss and improve or prevent health problems. .

As part of a medical obesity management program developed by a physician, it is important to perform regular exercise. For older adults regular exercise is effective therapy for stress reduction, sleep disorders, depression and anxiety. Your physician should be an important part of your pre-exercise prescription to examine cardiac risk, possible limitations, and contraindications to increased physical activity (14).

Colon Cancer

Colon cancer is cancer of the large intestine in the lower part of the digestive system. Rectal cancer is cancer involving the last several inches of the digestive system. Together the two types of cancers are referred to as colorectal cancers.

There have been several studies that have examined the relationship between colon cancer and physical activity. Most of these studies have shown a 30-50% colon cancer risk reduction in the most active groups compared to those who are sedentary (15), (16), (17), and (18).

In addition to maintaining a healthy weight, it is important to maintain a healthy diet and exercise most days of the week. If you've been sedentary, the doctor may recommend starting slowly and build up to increased physical activity or exercise.

Fall Prevention and Aging

It is estimated that one of three people over the age of 65 fall each year and one in every ten falls result in serious injury requiring medical care or hospitalization. Some of the more common injuries include hip, shoulder, and wrist fractures. Injuries may also occur to the brain, (called closed head injuries) as a result of striking the head on a hard surface. Closed head injuries can be particularly traumatic and can lead to death. Once a person has fallen, fear of future falls can lead to decreased physical activity and social isolation. Unless addressed, the "fear of falling cycle" can then lead to a further decrease in physical activity which places the individual at even greater risk of future falls.

Older people who are sedentary are at greater risk for falls. It has been shown that moving from being sedentary to at least moderately active can reduce the risk of hip fractures by 20-40% (19). Although many programs of exercise and increased physical activity have components of fall prevention built-in, fall prevention activities can also be performed independently. For example, activities such as standing at the kitchen counter on one foot and then the other enhance balance capabilities.

When designing a physical activity or exercise program be sure to include balance activities. To be most beneficial, balance activities should be performed 2-3 times a week. If poor balance is already a concern, or you are nervous about attempting exercise or have certain types of medical conditions, request your doctor suggest a health care professional provide initial balance training.

Exercise, Quality of Life and Functional Status

Studies regarding physical activity and quality of life consistently demonstrate an association between physical activity and perceived health, life satisfaction, decreased mood disturbance and life enjoyment (20), (21), (22). In general, older adults who participate in exercise on most days of the week will have better physical functioning than older persons who are periodically active or who are inactive. When facing a functional decline, physical activity is clearly better than no activity for protection against a functional decline. For those identified as being at risk for a functional decline regular exercise therapy should be incorporated as a part of the prescribed medical treatment.

Chapter Summary

This chapter discussed the importance of physical activity and exercise to manage and prevent healthcare problems. Physical activity is defined as performing activities that help get the body moving. Exercise is a form of physical activity but more structured so that activities are repetitive or concentrated on specific tasks.

It has been demonstrated that increasing physical activity and performing exercise have health benefits even if you have a health care problem. Some of the problems that exercise can help address include difficulty getting out of bed, standing, and walking. Regular exercise and increased physical activity also have important preventative aspects as well. Some of the problems exercise and increased physical activity can address before onset include:

Helping you retain the ability to do the things you want to do and enjoy.

Keep you on your feet by lowering your risk for falls and injury.

Help to prevent and manage diseases such as diabetes, heart disease, obesity, and colon cancer.

Lower the risk of stroke and improve blood pressure.

Increase physical strength and fitness by slowing the rate of loss of muscle mass

Improve you over-all sense of well-being.

Moving forward, the benefits obtained from implementing a physical activity and exercise program will depend upon three elements;

1. Your healthcare starting point,

2. The type of program selected and,

3. The effort and consistency you demonstrate in performance.

There are many exercises and activities to choose from. The next several chapters will address the best type of exercises and activities to perform and how to get started on a program you can enjoy.

Chapter 3

What to do Before Beginning to Exercise

Now that you recognize the importance increased physical activity and exercise will have upon your health it is time to make plans to safely get started. The purpose of this chapter is to help get organized and define an appropriate starting point. Once you have identified the important elements that need to be addressed then the process of increasing physical activity becomes much easier. This chapter focuses upon 2 important steps to get you started.

1. Start With Your Doctor

The exercises depicted in chapter five are typically safe for older adults who do not have serious health problems. They are specifically designed not to create stress on the body if performed slowly and properly. This is not to imply, however, you should attempt any increased physical activity or exercise without first speaking with your doctor. Why is it important to speak with your doctor before starting an increased activity and exercise program?

If you've had previous health care issues or have a current health problem, safety necessitates a doctor participate in the selection of the exercises to be performed. Your doctor may also insist on performing a physical examination, request special testing, or have a health professional such as a physical therapist help in the selection of the best exercises for you. For example, if you have an uncontrolled health problem, or have diabetes, heart disease, congestive heart failure (CHF), congestive obstructive pulmonary disease (COPD), arthritis, or have undergone back, hip, or knee surgery you'll need specialized direction regarding which activities are best for you.

On your next visit to your doctor ask the following question: "I have been reading a retirement, exercise, and fitness book and now understand the importance of exercise for improving my health." "The book discusses activities and exercises that are good for older adults." "Understanding my current health could you tell me where to begin?"

Other questions to ask the doctor may include:

- Are there activities or exercises that should be avoided (especially following surgery)?

- Should I avoid weights and resistance exercises? If so, for how long?

- With diabetes, what do I need to watch for when increasing my activities?

- With arthritis or recent injuries, are there certain types of exercises to avoid?

- Are there any medications that need to be changed as a result of increased activity?

It is important to tell your doctor if you have been experiencing chest pain or other cardiac symptoms, have an uncontrolled medical issue, a history of blood clots, or high blood pressure. Some other issues or symptoms to discuss with the doctor include:

- Dizziness or shortness of breath.
- A hernia.

- An infection or fever.
- Unexplained weight loss.
- Joint swelling.
- Leg sores that are slow to heal or will not heal.
- Issues with bleeding.
- A detached retina or recent eye surgery.

Your doctor understands the importance increased physical activity and exercise has upon health. When embarking upon a program of exercise, your doctor will be an invaluable resource helping to outline the best activities to perform and, thereby, reducing the potential risk of injury. The best advice before beginning any program of physical activity or exercise is to consult with your doctor.

2. Set Goals

One of the most important components of a plan to improve health is deciding what you want to accomplish. Some older adults believe deciding what to accomplish and establishing goals is difficult. The reason it can be difficult is because looking into the future and trying to decide what needs to be accomplished requires planning. As you will see, however, planning and setting goals may not be all that strenuous as compared to sustaining program commitment.

The issue most older people struggle with is sustaining commitment to a program of physical activity and exercise. To sustain lasting commitment to improved fitness requires behavioral change. As is well known, changing behavior is seldom easy to do. For example, it is not uncommon for 80-90% of people who make a "new year's resolution" to fail by the end of the first month.

It is not that the resolution was a bad idea. Typically a resolution will fail because not enough planning was done to modify behavior so commitment could be sustained. Planning and setting good goals is an essential foundational component to sustaining a lasting behavioral change and commitment to long term performance.

Setting Short Term Goals

Goal setting is a personal process. Although you can ask for others for assistance with setting goals the final determination is up to you. The purpose of this section of the book is to help identify activities that you'll find enjoyable and that will result in improved fitness from long term commitment.

When developing goals, the first decision to be made is when do you want to perform the activity and where it will be performed? For example, if you decide you want to walk increased distances outside, will walking be better in the morning or afternoon? Or if you want to exercise with a friend, what are the times available when the two of you can meet? Examples of short term goals that cover a period of 1-2 months include:

- I will increase my distance (or time) of walking to reach 5 blocks (or 30 minutes) at the end of 4 weeks.

- I will perform 1 set of 6 exercises with 10-15 repetitions (from Chapter 5) 15 minutes each day for 4 weeks.

In the early weeks of your fitness program, goals can be set at an easier level to help get started. For example, the goal of walking could start out with 5-10 minutes and be gradually progressed to 30 minutes. Remember, it is important to tailor the goal specifically to meet your need. The better the goal is defined the better the chance it will be accomplished.

Goals that are written-down are the ones most likely to be accomplished. Appendix 1 provides an opportunity to write down short and long term goals. Once goals are established, you can record activities completed on Appendix 2 and Appendix 3.

Setting Long Term Goals

Long term goals will reflect where you want to be in six months or a year. For example, the short term goal of being able to increase walking distances could lead to a long term goal such as:

- As a result of exercise and physical activity I will lose 10 pounds in 6 months from today.

- I will increase from my strength and distances of waking to a quarter of a mile to make it possible for me to help my daughter coach a little league softball team.

- I will increase my exercises from 1 set of 20 repetitions of 6 different exercises to the point where I can perform 3 sets of 20 repetitions of 10 different exercises (from Chapter 5) 3 days a week.

When establishing long term goals, make sure they are designed to personally to accommodate you. For example, select an activity that permits you to make an impact in another area of life. In your effort to improve your health are there areas where, with over-all improved fitness, you could volunteer? Success with long term fitness goals is best when celebrated with the ability to do something new at the end. Other factors to consider when setting goals and making fitness a priority include:

- Choose activities that appeal to you.

- Always take time to record your progress. Recording progress can act as positive feedback regarding performance.

- For the next few months, make increased physical activity a life "top priority." Set-aside a time each day and make it an "appointment" to complete the program of exercise and activity. Do everything possible not to skip those appointments.

- Make each exercise and activity enjoyable to perform. Avoid starting-out with too many exercises, too much weight to lift, or the use of too much resistance. A program that is too difficult could result in injury and commitment to performance could suffer.

- If you find certain types of music motivating or enjoyable while exercising then use them. If you like to watch sports while exercising then plan your program when you can exercise at the same time the events are televised.

Chapter Summary

A visit to your doctor is the first place to start when considering increasing your physical activity or performing an exercise program. Your doctor can provide the direction needed to ensure increasing physical activity is the right thing for you and help to decide activities and exercises that are safe.

If your doctor recommends a physical therapist to help design and implement a program, meet with a therapist that will tailor an exercise program to meet your physical fitness needs. As you become comfortable with your fitness program, your doctor may suggest you meet with the therapist again to design a more advanced exercise program that provides a greater fitness challenge.

Chapter 4

What are the Best Exercises for Me?

Older adults often report that participation in regular exercise and remaining physically active has little appeal. The reason behind limited appeal centers-around the belief that exercise, in order to be effective, must be performed in a gym. It is also a commonly held belief that exercise must be difficult or painful to perform in order to obtain any lasting benefit. These beliefs are not true.

This chapter focuses upon the identification of the four categories of exercise most beneficial to older adults. The four areas of exercise include: endurance, strength, balance, and flexibility. Each of these exercise areas are reviewed with recommendations regarding how seniors can identify opportunities to make exercise enjoyable. The chapter establishes a foundation for understanding that no one is too old or too frail to gain benefits from exercise and increased physical activity. Understanding that everyone, regardless of age, can obtain health benefits from exercise and physical activity helps in preparation for the next step. The next step involves making plans to get started!

The Four Types of Exercise

There are four types of exercise that are beneficial to perform for successful aging and fitness. The types are: **endurance, strength, balance, and flexibility.** Each of these will be discussed along with recommendations and examples for increasing safety with implementation.

1. Endurance Activities

Endurance exercises are activities designed to increase your heart rate and respiration over a period of time. Endurance exercises are helpful in delaying or preventing diseases such as colon cancer, heart disease, and diabetes. Endurance exercises include such activities as; jogging, swimming, playing tennis, walking, riding a bike, walking on a treadmill, or climbing stairs or hills.

The important aspect to remember with endurance activities is to build up endurance gradually. If you have been inactive for a while it may be necessary to start with 5 minutes or less of activity. Over time, however, the goal could be to work-up to 30 minutes of an activity. The goal of reaching 30 minutes of activity may not be for everyone. Setting realistic goals is essential and, to be effective, should take into account your current health status.

When performing endurance activities you must respond to the messages your body provides to you. Endurance exercises should not make you light headed, dizzy, cause chest pain, or present a feeling of heartburn. When you are performing endurance activities you should not struggle to breath or have such shortness of breath that makes it is difficult to talk.

Endurance activities often make you sweat but you may not feel thirsty. If you are sweating due to exercise, take time to have some water to avoid dehydration. If you have been advised by your doctor to limit your fluid intake then check with your doctor before increasing levels of fluid intake. Limiting fluid intake may be especially important to people who have been diagnosed with congestive heart failure or have kidney disease.

Creating a record of your endurance activities is essential to monitoring progress. Start out easy with the specific activity and, as you feel you can, increase the activity to the point where you can participate in that activity for 30 minutes several days per week. Figure 1 demonstrates how you can record your progress. Appendix 2 includes a weekly recording chart that can be repeatedly used over several weeks and months.

Week of 9/15	Sunday	Monday	Tuesday
Walking outside	Yes	Yes	Rained all day
Length of time	10 minutes	12 minutes	None

Figure 1. A record of daily endurance activities. On days where the activity cannot be completed, record the reason. The results may be shared with you doctor.

2. Strengthening Exercises

One of the greatest challenges facing older adults is maintaining strength. After the age of 50 years, it is understood that strength decreases more than 10% with each decade of life. Even small decreases in muscle strength can make it difficult to stand-up from a chair, climbing stairs, and can place you at increased risk for falls. For those reasons preventing or reversing muscle weakness must be a priority for older adults.

To increase strength you will need to perform resistive exercises. These types of exercise can include lifting weights, resistance bands, weighted objects that you can create, or things you have around the house. It is certainly acceptable to perform exercises in a gym but the focus of this book is upon the opportunity you have to exercise in the privacy of your own home.

To be effective, strengthening exercises should be performed a minimum of 2 times per week. Sessions should last approximately 30 minutes. It is important to start out either using no weight or as little as 1-2 pounds. When using resistive bands begin at lower resistance levels and gradually progress upward in difficulty.

Injuries to older adults due to weight lifting are infrequent as long as careful attention is paid to using lighter weights, following the correct lifting technique, and not increasing the use of heavier weights too soon. For safety purposes it advisable to use very light weights for the first two weeks. Other recommendations include:

- Begin your exercise program using a level of weight that you can lift 8-10 times. Over the next week or so, progress to where you can lift the same weight 15 times.

- Once 15 repetitions becomes easy then add a second set of repetitions and repeat the activity until you can perform 2 sets
  of 15-20 repetitions. When 2 sets of 15-20 repetitions becomes easy you can add more weight and begin again at performing 8-10 repetitions.

This process can be repeated to the point where the exercise is a challenge to perform but remains safe and not strenuous. At any point where exercise becomes too hard, reduce the weight to the previous level and remain at that weight. Do not resume using increased weight levels until the former resistance becomes very easy to perform.

Consider following the 7 second rule for lifting weights. It should take you three seconds to push the weight into place, hold that position for one second, and take another 3 seconds to return the weight to the starting position. Injuries occur when weights are jerked into position or dropped too quickly. Make it your goal to control the resistance and your speed of movement.

If you have a medical condition, have recently been hospitalized, or had surgery, discuss with your doctor or surgeon what type of exercises you are allowed to perform. Depending upon your medical condition, it is not uncommon for your doctor to recommend physical or occupational therapy to get you started in the right direction before proceeding on your own.

If you have problems with balance or have weakness in the legs, you may exercise in a chair. For safety purposes, you can accomplish the same objectives performing exercises in a chair and not have to be concerned with falling and sustaining an injury.

Expect for your muscles to be sore for the first week or two as you accommodate to the increased activity. You may also experience some fatigue. Once the program is established your body should accommodate as long as you slowly increase the level of weights or resistance-band training you are performing.

Breathing in a regular pattern is essential for proper weight lifting. Always remember to breathe out as you lift the weight and breathe in as you lower the weight to the starting position. Be patient, it may take time to develop this breathing pattern as you also follow the 7 second rule for lifting weights.

If your goal to exercise in the privacy of your home that is certainly an available option. In order to do so your doctor may suggest you see a physical or occupational therapist for recommendations on specific exercises (some of which may not be included in this book) that can be performed in the home. Some low cost examples for creating weights in the home include:

- Fill plastic containers (milk jugs or soda bottles) with marbles, sand, or water. Weigh them on a scale or use one pound cans to estimate the weight of the container.

- Fill a sock with rocks or marbles and tightly secure the open end.

- Use resistive bands or tubing. Resistive bands come in several colors and the colors are designed to identify how difficult the resistance will be. A physical or occupational therapist can help identify the best starting point to begin with color selection.

3. Balance Exercises

Balance is a complex function that involves several systems in the body. Maintaining balance is a coordinated process that includes the eyes, the inner ear, and the sensation information your brain obtains through your feet and muscles. All systems need to work together to ensure that you are able to remain up-right and lower the risk of falling.

To be effective, especially with aging, balance exercises need to be performed throughout the week. They can be included as part of a strengthening program or can be performed separately. Examples of different ways to challenge balance include:

- While standing, increase or decrease your base of support by standing with the feet apart, feet close together, with one foot in
  front of the other in a heel to toe position, or standing on one leg.
- Turning the head side-to-side while placing the feet close together, far apart, or while standing heel-to-toe.
- Brushing teeth while standing on one foot.
- With a counter-top to hold-on-to, close your eyes. Rotate your head side-to-side with eyes closed.
- Walking in figure eight patterns.
- Increasing and decreasing to speed at which you walk.
- Toss a ball into the air while walking.
- Participating in water aerobics.

In the exercise and balance section of this book you will see exercises directed toward the muscles in the ankle, trunk, thigh, and hip. For fall prevention purposes, these muscles are vital for performing functional activities such as getting in and out of the shower, standing up from a bed or chair and walking, making safe turns, and going up and down a step or stairs. Many balance activities and exercises can be performed as often you would like and in any setting as long as you use a solid chair, wall, or counter-top for safety and support.

4. Flexibility Exercises

As aging progresses many seniors report reduced freedom of movement in the performance of daily activities. For example, it may become more difficult to get dressed, reach objects on the shelf or pick them up from the floor, or to put on and take-off pants, shoes or socks. Flexibility exercises, also known as stretching exercises are designed to retain the flexibility needed to perform daily activities and maximize independence. Neck, upper extremity and trunk flexibility is especially important for safe automobile driving. Flexibility is needed to turn your head and reposition the body for turns or for backing into or out of parking spaces.

Flexibility exercises are easy to incorporate into an exercise program. They can be incorporated as part of the warm-up and cool-down parts of the program. Performing flexibility exercises will not increase strength or endurance. In the flexibility section of chapter five you will see exercises that can performed prior to strengthening, endurance, or balance activities. Some important things to remember with flexibility exercises include:

- Always perform the stretch slowly. Proceed with the stretch as far as possible being careful to avoid pain. Once in the position, try to maintain the stretch for 10-15 seconds before slowly letting-off.

- If you have had surgery, check with your doctor before

beginning any attempt to increase flexibility. There are specific types of surgery where flexibility exercises should not be performed until full healing has occurred.

- Avoid performing a "bounce" stretch. All stretches should be performed slowly with special emphasis on holding the stretch position once it is reached. Performing bounce stretches do not provide the long term results that can be obtained by slow stretches and increase the risk of injury to the muscles being stretched.

- Remember to avoid holding your breath. Holding your breath should be avoided with all exercises but normal breathing should be maintained with flexibility exercises. To avoid holding your breath while stretching speak out loud or sing or hum a song to yourself.

- If you are experiencing sharp or stabbing pain while performing a stretch or the pain lingers into the next day, you are pushing the stretch position too far. When in doubt, reduce the stretch so that pain is eliminated.

- Avoid the "locked position" in all joints that are being stretched. The goal is to have a small amount of bend in the joint but not to have excessive stress being applied to the joint. Also, if you have had any joint surgery check with the surgeon to determine if stretching involving the joint should be performed.

Chapter Summary

The four types of exercise to perform for successful aging and fitness are: endurance, strength, balance, and flexibility. The benefits to performing each of these exercises far out-weigh the risks of potential injury. As a matter-of-fact, you stand a bigger risk of doing damage to your health by not increasing physical activity rather than from increasing your physical activity.

In the beginning stages of increasing your level of physical activity you may experience increased discomfort or fatigue but that should lessen as you begin to accommodate to the new program. The key is to go slowly and perform the activities that you find are comfortable for you.

It is unlikely the new activity and exercise program you implement will be exactly like the type performed by friends or family. Having a personalized program that is different from what other people perform is 100% okay.

The key to a successful program is to participate in activities you enjoy, that are safe and effective for you, and that you are most likely to continue performing. Following an individualized philosophy to increasing your fitness levels will likely provide you with the greatest success.

Chapter 5

Home Based Exercises

A complete home based program of physical activity and exercise should focus upon activities that challenge your body in the four areas as mentioned in this book. The four areas are:

Strength

Flexibility

Endurance

Balance

This chapter provides sample exercises that address each of these four areas along with written recommendations regarding how to perform each activity safely. There are many other types of exercises not shown in this book that your doctor or physical therapist may suggest you perform.

Always follow the recommendations that are provided by your physician and physical therapist. Their recommendations for exercise will be based solely upon a thorough understanding of your health history and what type of physical activity and exercise will be best for you. To help monitor exercise performance, an exercise tracking chart has been included in Appendix 3.

Strength - Upper Extremities*

Purpose: To strengthen the shoulders and arms to make activities such as reaching over-head, lifting, and carrying easier and safer to do.

1. Over-head Arm Press*

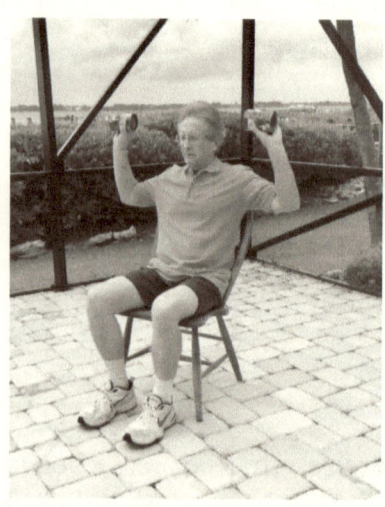 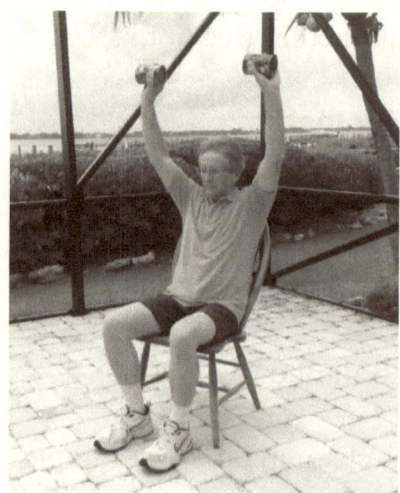

1. Perform seated.
2. Feet flat on the floor.
3. Weights slightly above shoulder height.
4. Elbows bent.
5. Raise arms while breathing out.
6. Hold in the up position for 1-2 seconds.
7. Breath-in while lowering the weights.
8. Repeat 10-15 times.
9. Rest as needed.
10. Record exercise performance.

*Obtain physician approval prior to performing.

2. Front Arm Raise*

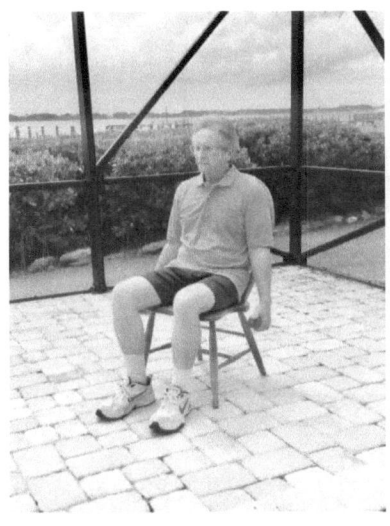 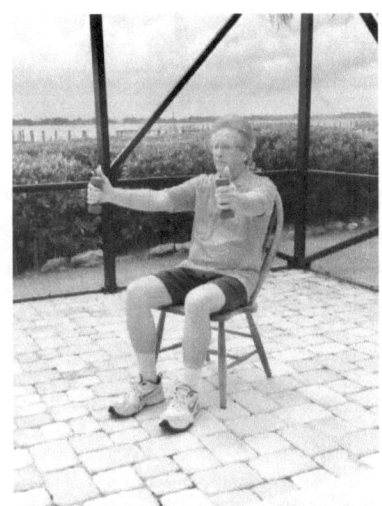

1. Perform seated.
2. Feet flat on the floor.
3. Weights at Side.
4. Elbows slightly bent.
5. Raise arms while breathing out (with thumbs up).
6. Hold in up position for 1-2 seconds
7. Breath-in while lowering the weights.
8. Repeat 10-15 times.
9. Rest as needed.
10. Record exercise performance.

*Obtain physician approval prior to performing.

3. Alternating Arm Curl*

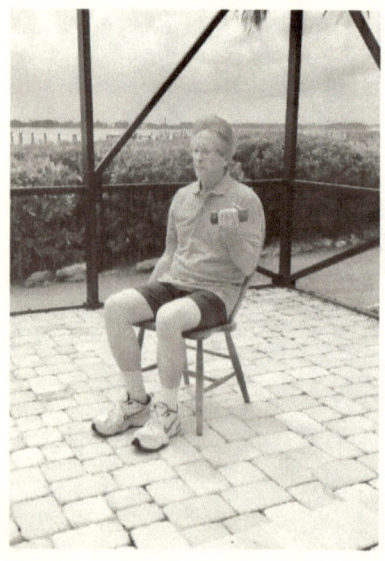 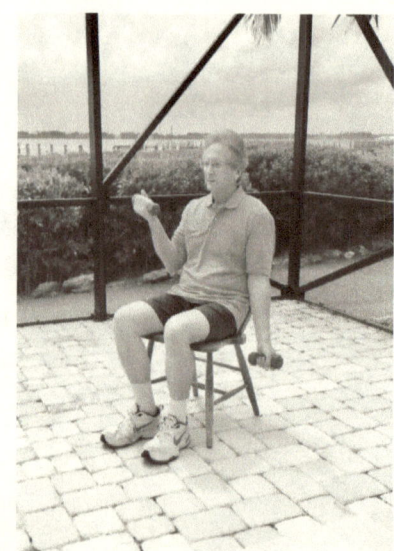

1. Perform seated.
2. Feet flat on the floor.
3. Weights at side.
4. Elbows straight.
5. Raise weights while breathing out.
6. Hold in up position for 1-2 seconds.
7. Breath-in while lowering the weights.
8. Repeat 10-15 times.
9. Rest as needed.
10. Record exercise performance.

*Obtain physician approval prior to performing.

4. Rowing With Resistance Band*

Resistance bands come in many colors with each type providing a different level of resistance. Start with an easy level band and gradually increase the level difficulty as desired.

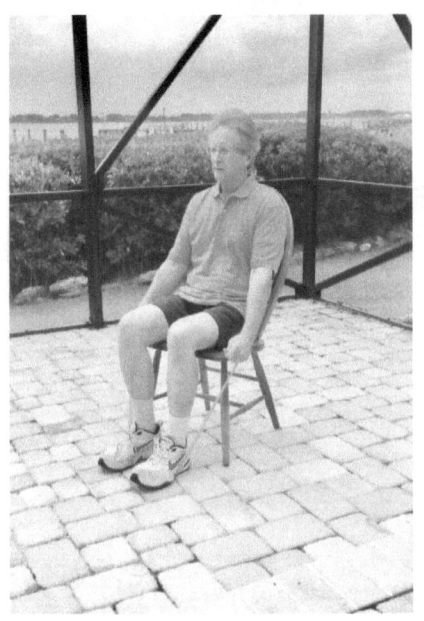 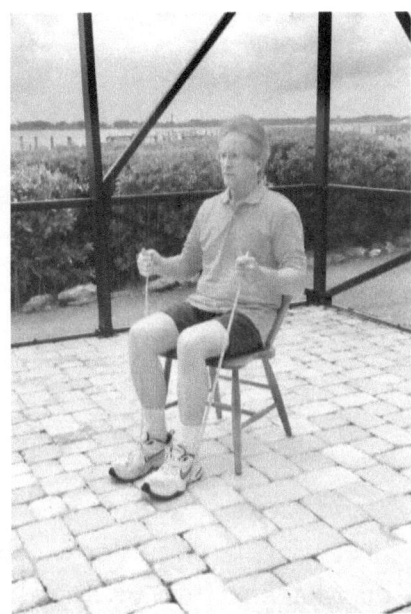

1. Perform seated.
2. Feet flat on the floor.
3. Band centered under both feet.
4. Elbows bent.
5. Row up and back while breathing out.
6. Hold in position for 1-2 seconds
7. Breath in while rowing forward.
8. Repeat 10-15 times.
9. Rest as needed.
10. Record exercise performance.

*Obtain physician approval prior to performing.

5. Wall Push-up*

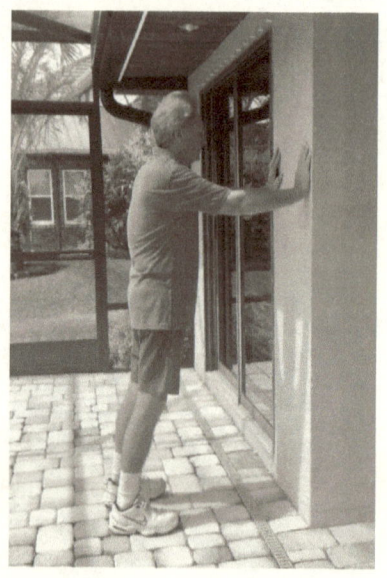 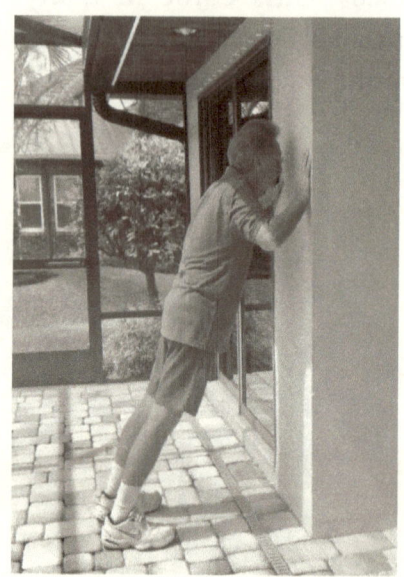

1. Stand facing a wall.
2. Feet apart to shoulder width.
3. Feet back slightly greater than arms-length to wall.
4. Lean into wall, palms flat, keep trunk straight.
5. While breathing in, slowly touch nose to wall.
6. Hold 1-2 seconds.
7. While breathing out, push yourself to the start position.
8. Repeat 10-15 times.
9. Rest as needed.
10. Record exercise performance.

*Obtain physician approval prior to performing.

Strength – Lower Extremities*

Purpose: To strengthen the legs, making activities such as walking, going-up and down stairs, getting in and out of a chair, and on-and-off a toilet seat easier and safer to do.

1. Knee Extension*

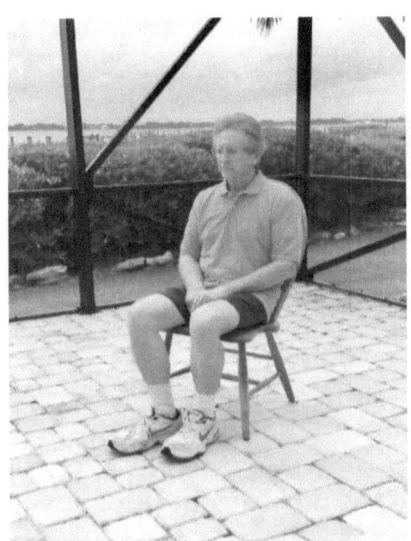 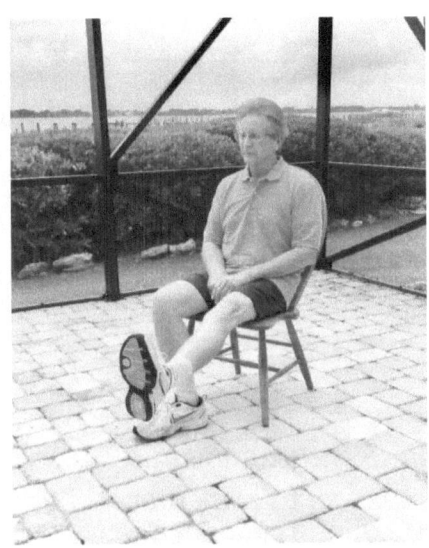

1. Perform seated.
2. Feet flat on the floor.
3. Breath-out and slowly extend leg in front to straight.
4. Pull toes and foot toward you. Hold 2 seconds.
5. Relax foot and toes.
6. While breathing out, slowly lower leg back to the beginning position.
7. Perform with the opposite leg.
8. Repeat 10-15 times.
9. Rest as needed.
10. Record exercise performance.

*Obtain physician approval prior to performing.

2. Hip Extension*

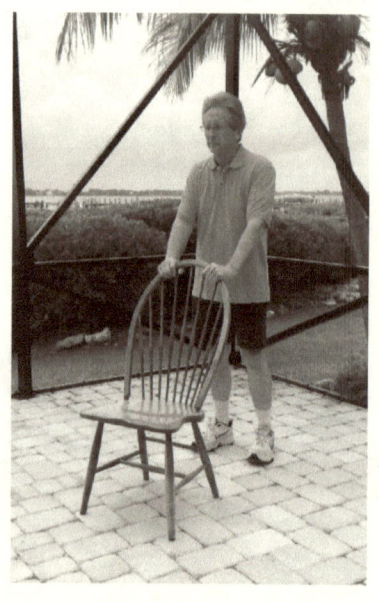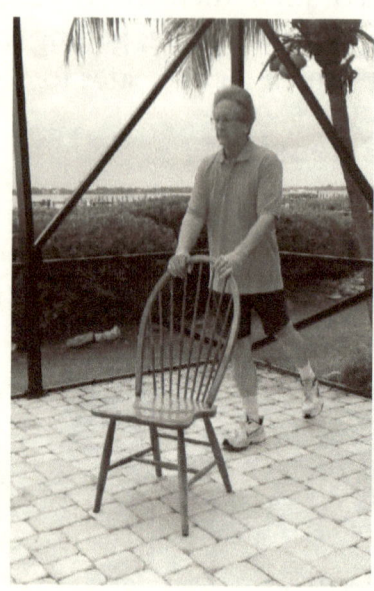

1. Perform Standing.
2. Hold-on to a counter-top or very sturdy chair (both hands).
3. Keep both knees straight.
4. While breathing out, move one leg back.
5. Keep the leg moved back in the straight position.
6. Hold 1-2 seconds.
7. While breathing in, slowly lower leg to start position.
8. Repeat 10-15 times.
9. Rest as needed.
10. Record exercise performance.

*Obtain physician approval prior to performing.

3. Hip Abduction*

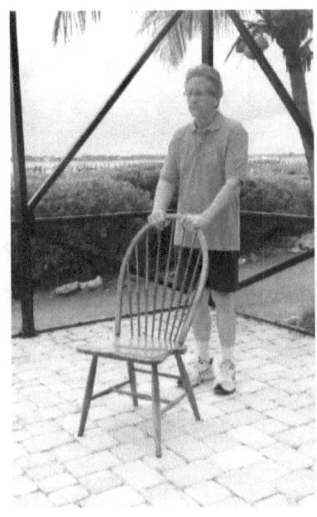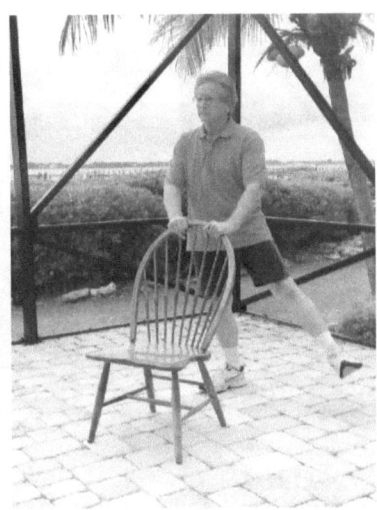

1. Perform Standing.
2. Hold-on to a counter-top or very sturdy chair.
3. Keep both knees straight.
4. While breathing out, move one leg out sideways.
5. Keep the toes forward and leg in the straight position.
6. Hold 1-2 seconds.
7. While breathing in, slowly lower leg to start position.
8. Repeat 10-15 times.
9. Rest as needed.
10. Record exercise performance.

*Obtain physician approval prior to performing.

4. Sit-to-Stand *

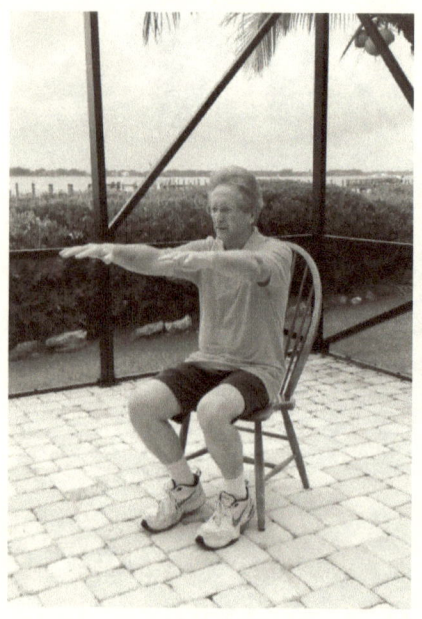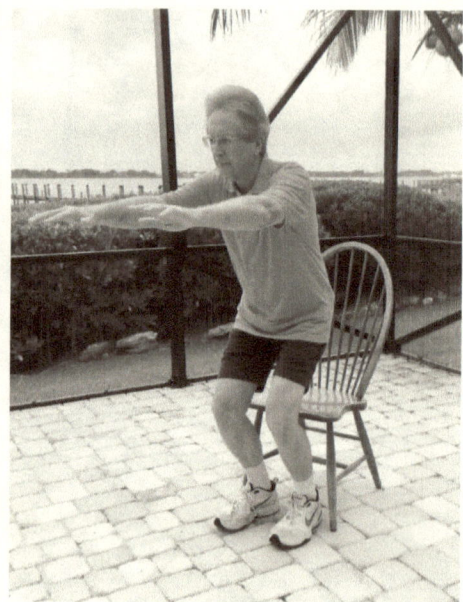

1. On a very sturdy chair, begin from the seated upright position.
2. Heels positioned at front edge of the chair.
3. Arms forward.
4. While breathing out, slowly stand up.
5. Once standing, keep the posture straight as possible.
6. Remain standing 5 seconds.
7. While breathing in, slowly lower yourself to start position.
8. Repeat 10-15 times.
9. Rest as needed.
10. Record exercise performance.

*Obtain physician approval prior to performing.

5. Heel Rise*

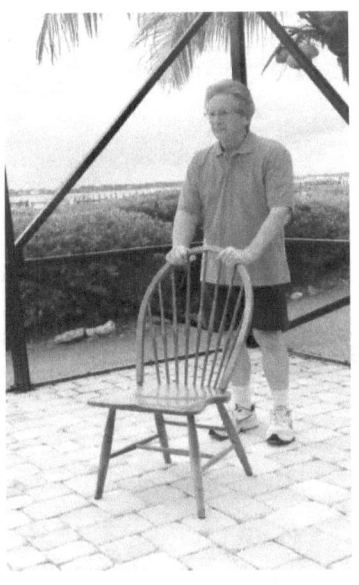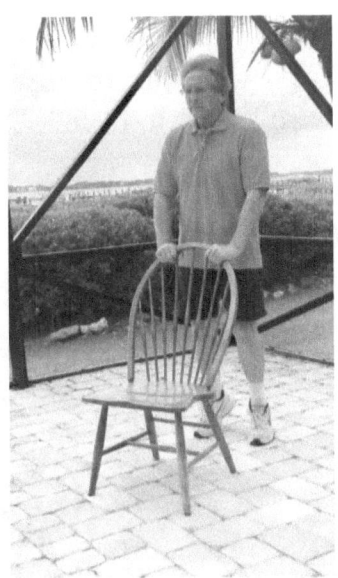

1. Perform Standing.
2. Hold-on to a counter-top or very sturdy chair.
3. Keep both knees straight.
4. While breathing out, move onto tip-toes.
5. Keep posture as straight as possible.
6. Hold 1-2 seconds.
7. While breathing in, slowly lower leg to start position.
8. Repeat 10-15 times.
9. Rest as needed.
10. Record exercise performance.

*Obtain physician approval prior to performing.

Flexibility*

Purpose: To keep yourself limber providing increased freedom of movement, lessen the opportunity for injury, and making every-day activities easier and safer to do.

1. Seated Chest Stretch*

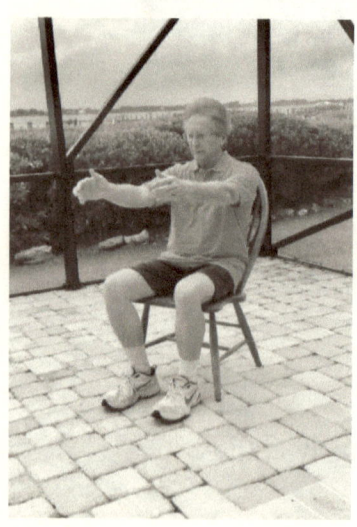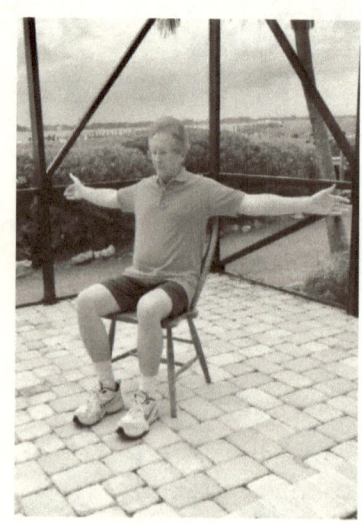

1. Perform seated.
2. Keep feet flat on the floor.
3. Move arms out to side, elbows straight, thumbs-up.
4. While breathing out, raise arms toward the side.
5. Keep posture as straight.
6. When reaching fully-out-the-side, hold 1-2 seconds.
7. While breathing in, slowly return to the start position.
8. Repeat 10-15 times.
9. Rest as needed.
10. Record exercise performance.

*Obtain physician approval prior to performing.

2. Seated Back Stretch*

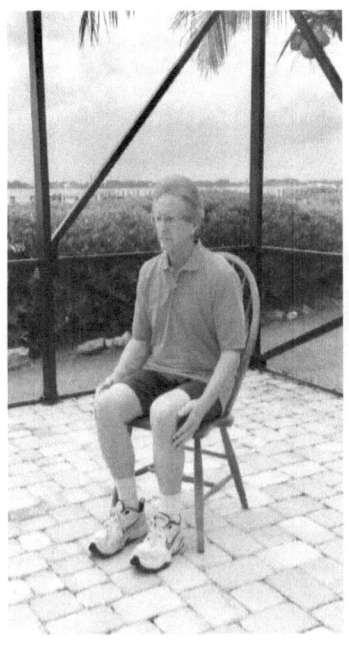 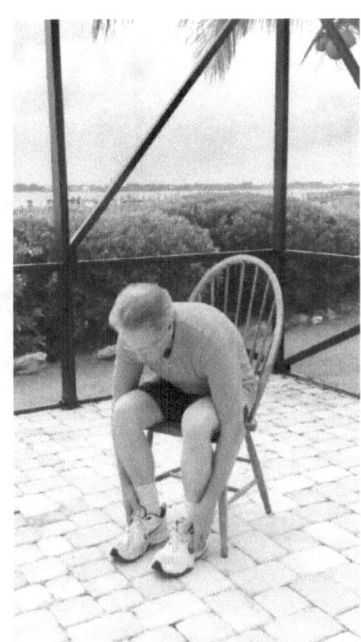

1. Perform seated.
2. Keep feet flat on the floor.
3. Move arms out to side of knees.
4. While breathing out, slowly lean forward while hands move along
    out-side of calves.
5. Allow head to flex forward as you move downward.
6. When reaching as low as comfortable, hold 15-30 seconds.
7. While breathing in, slowly return to the starting position.
8. Repeat 3-5 times.
9. Rest as needed.
10. Record exercise performance.

*Obtain physician approval prior to performing.

3. Seated Trunk Rotation*

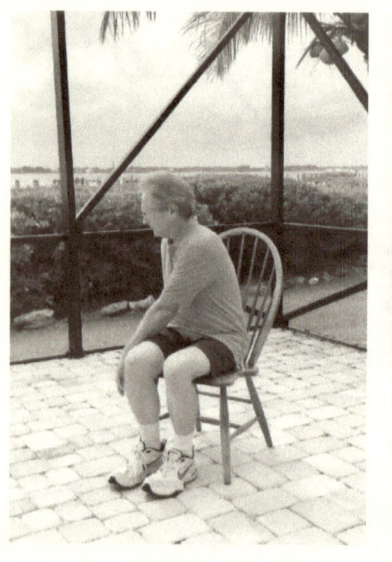 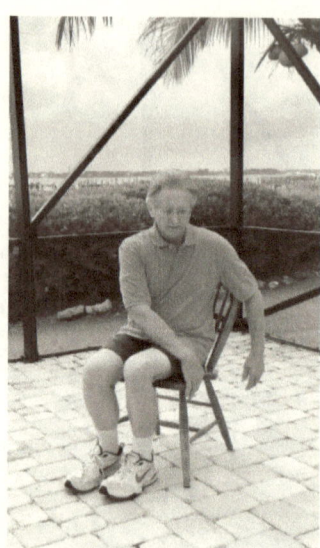

1. Perform seated.
2. Keep feet flat on the floor
3. Move arms to a comfortable position.
4. While breathing out, slowly rotate to the right.
5. When reaching as far as comfortable, hold 5-10 seconds.
6. Return to center while breathing in.
7. Repeat rotation to the left side.
8. Repeat 3-5 times to each side.
9. Rest as needed.
10. Record exercise performance.

*Obtain physician approval prior to performing.

4. Posterior Leg Stretch*

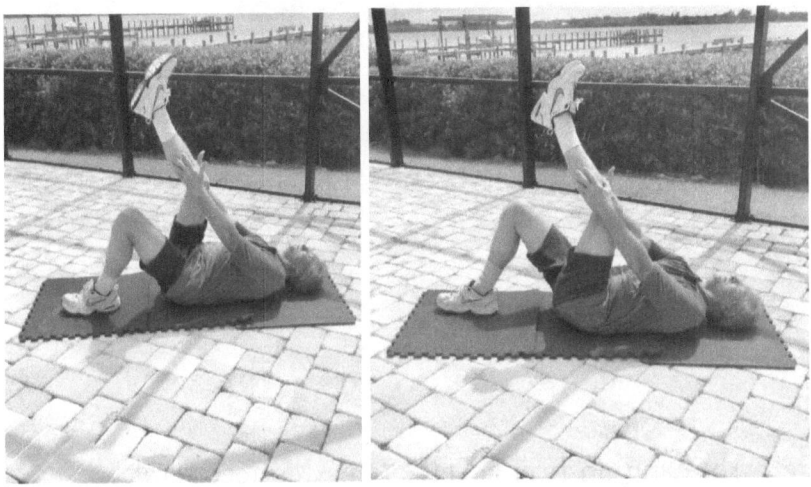

1. Perform lying on firm surface (a bed is acceptable).
2. Keep shoulders and back flat on the surface.
3. While breathing out, begin with right leg, keeping it slightly bent, raise toward the chest.
4. Use hands to pull leg gently toward the chest.
5. When reaching a comfortable position, hold 5-10 seconds.
6. Breath in while returning to the surface of the bed.
7. Repeat on the left side.
8. Repeat 3-5 times on each leg.
9. Rest as needed.
10. Record exercise performance.

*Obtain physician approval prior to performing.

4. Lower Back Stretch*

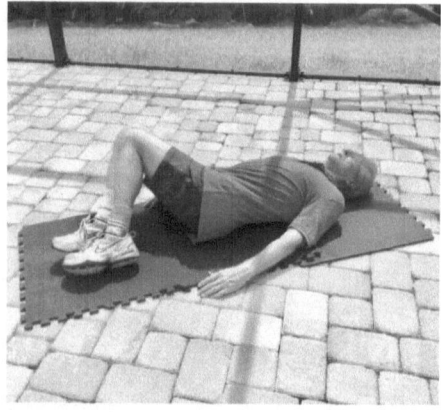 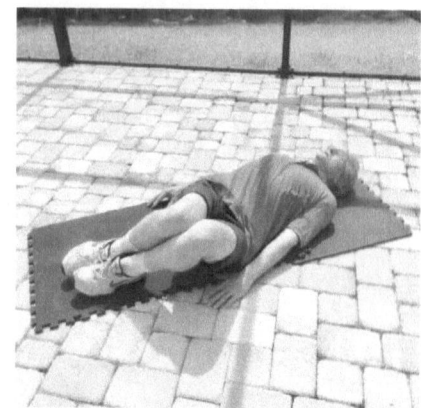

1. Perform lying on firm surface (a bed is acceptable).
2. Keep shoulders and back flat on the surface.
3. Bend knees to comfortable position.
4. While breathing out, begin lower trunk rotation to the right.
5. When reaching a comfortable position, hold 5-10 seconds.
6. Breath in while returning to the center position.
7. Repeat on the left side.
8. Repeat 3-5 times on each leg.
9. Rest as needed.
10. Record exercise performance.

*Obtain physician approval prior to performing.

5. Standing Calf Stretch*

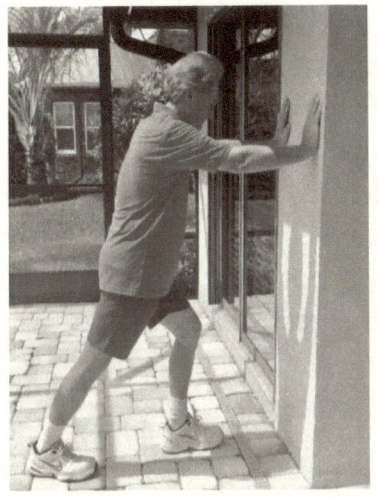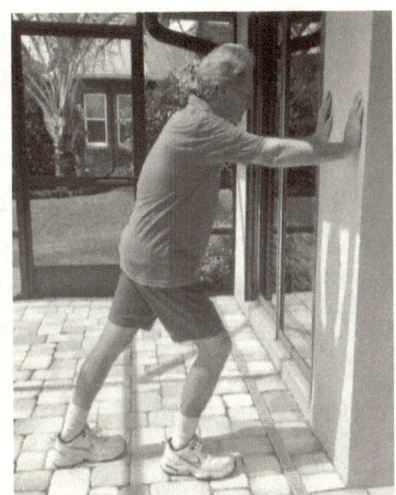

1. Stand facing a wall.
2. Place palms flat on the surface of the wall, shoulder height.
3. Place the right leg slightly back from left leg.
4. Keep the right heel on the floor and slightly bend the left knee while leaning forward. Breathe-out while performing the stretch.
5. When reaching a comfortable stretch position, hold 15-30 seconds.
6. Breath in while returning to the non-stretch position.
7. Repeat on the left side.
8. Repeat 3-5 times on each leg.
9. Rest as needed.
10. Record exercise performance.

*Obtain physician approval prior to performing.

Endurance Exercises

As we age our endurance for activities begins to decline. A decline in endurance may be seen as increased difficulty with day-to-day activities such as walking up-stairs, shopping, or performing activities around the home. The loss of endurance is a part of growing older but we can work to maintain or increase our stamina with aging.

Endurance exercises include activities that increase the heart rate and breathing rate over extended periods of time. If you have not been active for a long time you must work-up to an increased level of activity slowly. Performed on a regular basis, endurance exercises increase energy levels, improve fat metabolism, and help prevent heart disease.

Examples of Moderate Endurance Activities:

Bicycling
Walking on level surfaces
Cycling on a stationary bike
Mopping a floor.
Golf without a cart
Doubles tennis
Dancing
Volleyball

Examples of Vigorous Endurance Activities:

Hill or stair climbing
Bicycling up hill
Jogging
Hiking
Lap swimming
Singles tennis
Cross country skiing

Where and How to Begin Endurance Activities

Before beginning any endurance activity speak with your physician. Based upon your physical condition, your physician will be able to advise you how to listen to your body when it sends out signals you may be over-doing-it.

With endurance exercise, the goal is to build-up the activity level gradually. If you have been inactive for a long time it is perfectly acceptable to begin with as little as 5 minutes of activity and have as a goal to increase the time over several weeks or months. The goal should be to increase your endurance based activity from no less than 10 minutes a day to a total of 30 minutes a day on most days of the week.

Endurance Activity Safety Tips

1. **Always warm-up and cool down**. Before participation in any endurance activity, you should set-aside 5 minutes on both sides of the activity to warm-up and cool down. Warm-up and cool down activities could be as simple as mild stretching or walking to help prepare your body before and after the activity. Stretching before the activity helps reduce the opportunity for injury. Stretching afterwards helps keep you from experiencing post-activity muscle tightness and cramping.

2. **Watch for signs the activity is too intense**. No endurance activity should make you breath so hard or become so short of breath that you cannot talk. With any endurance activity it is abnormal to experience chest pain or pressure or experience dizziness.

3. **Wear good shoes.** Regardless of the endurance activity wear proper fitting shoes. A good fitting shoe helps support the foot and lessens the chances of injury. If you have circulatory issues in your feet or legs consult your physician regarding how to watch for changes in the skin. The endurance activity should not increase lower extremity pain or lead to the development of blisters or sores.

4. **Endurance activities and sweating**. Many endurance activities will increase sweating. The problem is, with increased aging, the body may not send out signals that it is time to drink water. This may eventually lead to dehydration. If your physician has requested you to control fluid intake consult with the physician regarding how much fluid you should have with an endurance activity.

In order to safely and effectively monitor the progress of your endurance activities, the results need to be recorded. Appendix 2 provides an opportunity for you to track daily progress in a format that can be shared with your physician.

Balance Exercises

One thing in life that can quickly change a retirement plan is a loss of balance and fall. It is important to recognize that falling is not considered a normal part of aging. Here is some important data regarding senior falls:

One in five falls causes a serious injury such as a broken bone or head injury.

Each year 800,000 patients are hospitalized because of a fall injury. Most often the hospitalization is because of a head injury or hip fracture.

Each year at least 300,000 elderly people are hospitalized for hip fractures.

More than 95% of hip fractures are caused by falling.

The risk of breaking a hip increases with aging.

Falling once doubles the chances of falling again.

There are exercises you can perform on a regular basis that will help lower the risk of falling. Regardless of whether you are trying to "maintain good balance health" or trying to correct a problem with balance, it is always best to start off with simple balance exercises.

Balance Exercises*

1. Single Limb Stance*

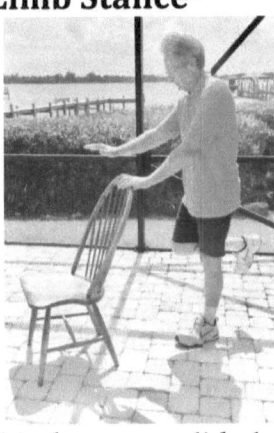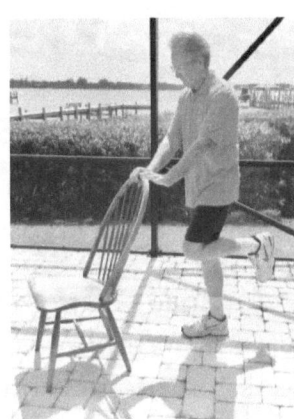

1. Stand behind a very solid chair or at a kitchen counter-top.
2. Place both hands on the chair.
3. Lift the right leg slightly off the floor and bend knee.
4. Slowly take the right hand off the back of the chair.
5. Hold the position, for 10-15 seconds.
6. Lower the right foot back to the start position and place the right hand back on the chair.
7. Repeat on the left side.
8. Repeat 3-5 times on each leg.
9. Rest as needed.
10. Record exercise performance.

*Obtain physician approval prior to performing. There are some medical conditions where this exercise will be 100% discouraged by your doctor.

2. The 12 to 6 Clock*

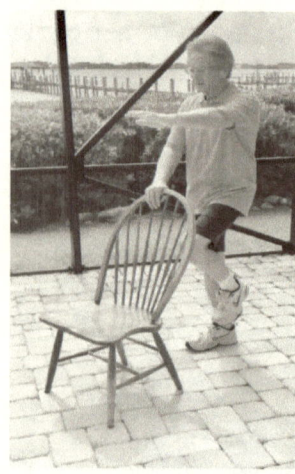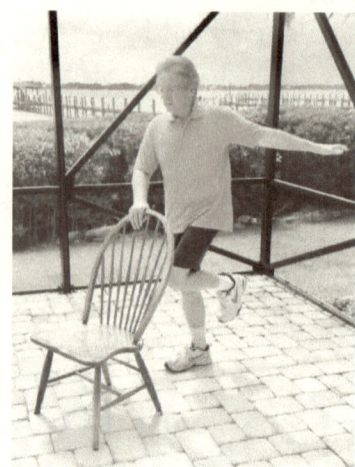

1. Stand behind a very solid chair or at a kitchen counter-top (the number 12 is directly in front of you and the number 6 is directly behind you). Look forward the entire time.
2. Place both hands on the chair.
3. Lift the left leg slightly off the floor.
4. Slowly take the left hand off the surface and extend your arm forward so it is pointing at the 12.
5. Hold the position, and then move the arm toward the number 3, and then the number 6. Return the arm to the number 3 and then number 12.
6. Lower the left foot back to the start position and place the left hand back on the chair.
7. Repeat on the left side.
8. Repeat 3-5 times on each leg.
9. Rest as needed.
10. Record exercise performance.

*Obtain physician approval prior to performing. There are some medical conditions where this exercise will be 100% discouraged by your doctor.

3. Back Leg Raise*

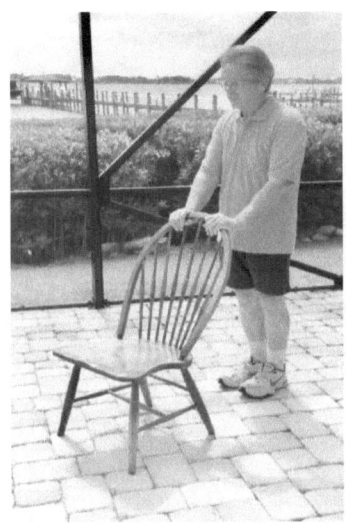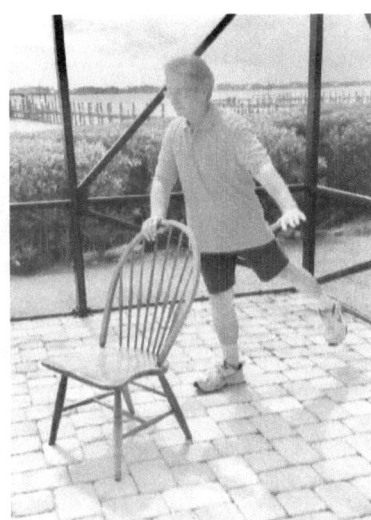

1. Stand behind a very solid chair or at a kitchen counter-top. Look forward the entire time.
2. Place both hands on the chair or counter-top.
3. Lift the left leg slightly off the floor and move it backwards while keeping the knee straight. Remove left hand from surface.
4. Avoid bending the knees.
5. Hold the position for 5 seconds.
6. Lower the left foot back to the start position.
7. Repeat on the right side.
8. Repeat 3-5 times on each leg.
9. Rest as needed.
10. Record exercise performance.

*Obtain physician approval prior to performing. There are some medical conditions where this exercise will be 100% discouraged by your doctor.

3. Side Leg Raise*

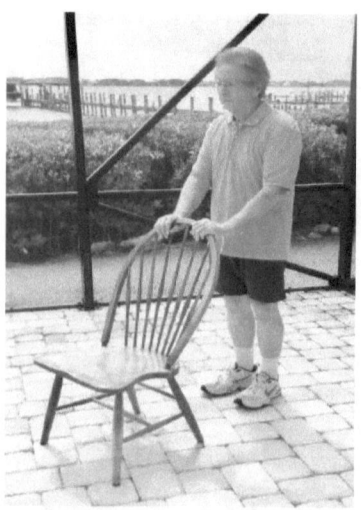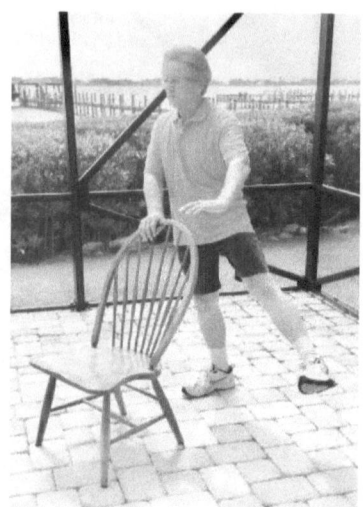

1. Stand behind a very solid chair or at a kitchen counter-top. Look forward the entire time.
2. Place both hands on the chair or counter-top.
3. Lift the left leg slightly off the floor and move it out sideways while keeping the knee straight. Remove left hand from surface.
4. Keep the back straight and the foot pointed forward.
5. Hold the position for 5 seconds.
6. Lower the left leg back to the start position.
7. Repeat on the right side.
8. Repeat 3-5 times on each leg.
9. Rest as needed.
10. Record exercise performance.

*Obtain physician approval prior to performing. There are some medical conditions where this exercise will be 100% discouraged by your doctor.

Chapter Summary

This chapter provided sample exercises that address each of these four areas of focus for those interested in improving personal fitness. The four areas of focus in this chapter were: **strength, endurance, flexibility, and balance.**

There are some medical conditions where exercise will be discouraged by your doctor. Before starting an exercise program review with your doctor all exercises you have an interest in performing. A professional will always make recommendations based upon an understanding of your health history and what type of physical activity and exercise best for you.

Chapter 6

Remaining Motivated to Exercise

One of the challenges faced by many who undertake the initiative to increase physical activity and exercise is motivation to keep the program going. This is not an uncommon problem even those who are truly committed to improving their level of fitness.

This chapter discusses some of the common reasons why physical activity programs are stopped and the best attitude to have for keeping activities going. Suggestions are provided that will be helpful for keeping you on the "exercise track" or getting you "back on track" if you have stopped your fitness efforts.

Some Reasons Why Physical Activity Programs Stop

People stop a program of increased physical fitness or exercise for any number of reasons. This is especially true once the program has been in place for a long period of time. What is most important to understand is why you stopped the program so that you can take appropriate steps to get going again. The following are some of the primary reasons why people stop an existing program:

1. A Change in Health - If you have recently had a healthcare episode that required hospitalization or have been ill due to other causes, you may not feel up to resuming the program you were previously performing. In order to get back-on-track you may need to resume the program at a lower level of activity. Based upon the type or severity of the recent illness, your doctor will be the primary

esource for directing when it is time to resume previous activity
evels.

2. A Change of Medication. Occasionally changes in medication
can impact your abilities to perform physical activities. For example, if
you have been placed on a new cardiac medication your doctor may
ask that you not be as physically active as you once were in order to
give your body time to accommodate to the new dosage. This may
also apply if you are taking medications for congestive heart failure
(CHF), congestive obstructive pulmonary disease (COPD), or
diabetes. Whenever there is a change in medication, or a change the
dosage of a medication, ask the doctor when previous activity levels
can safely be resumed.

3. A Change in Housing. If you have recently relocated to a new
living setting this change may upset the established routine. For
example, if you moved from your home to an assisted living facility
you may be on a new schedule that is much different than what you
had before. Take time to adjust to the new residential schedule and
then re-start your program once you have an understanding of how
the new location operates.

4. A Family Emergency. When someone close to you has a life
threatening emergency your schedule may be disrupted for several
weeks. During that time, and possibly for some time after the
emergency is resolved, previous exercises and activities may have to
be stopped. Always attend to the emergency without experiencing
guilt from stopping the program. It can be resumed once things are
back to normal.

5. This is Boring. For those new to increased physical activity or
for those who have been exercising for a while, it is important to
recognize that even the best program can become stale. When that
occurs make adjustments to the program to make it enjoyable. This

may include making changes in the location where the activities are performed, adding or changing music, or inviting someone to exercise with you. Additional suggestions are provided in the next section.

Renewing A Commitment to Physical Activity

If you have stopped or are thinking about stopping your physical activity and exercise program there are a few things you can do to keep yourself on-track. Consider the following to help renew your commitment:

1. Change-up the Activities – The next time you plan to go to the store set-aside increased time for walking. For example, rather than just go to one store in the mall, take time to walk increased distances inside the mall. Many malls also have a "mall walker program" that allows community residents the opportunity to walk inside the mall one hour before the stores open. Malls often have computed the distances so progress can be recorded.

2. Make the Program More Social - If your program has you exercising by yourself see if there are opportunities to exercise with others. The local recreation department may offer classes in yoga, Tai Chi, balance classes, or aerobic activities. You may also be able to join a gym with a month-to-month membership to keep costs low. Many local gyms also offer programs designed for older adults.

3. Try a Different Approach - For a month try to perform different activities outside of the residence. For example, walk in the park, ride a bike, or volunteer for community activities that require physical activity. Use stairs if they are available and walk to close-by stores rather than driving or riding a bus.

4. Review the Activities You've Been Performing – If you have a program that is focused on just one or two types of activity then examine opportunities to do other things. For example, if the current program has focused on endurance and strength then look for opportunities to address balance and flexibility. Adding new or different types of exercises is effective for helping to maintain exercise commitment.

Chapter Summary

It is important to understand there will be times when you simply don't want to exercise, or the surroundings are not available that will allow you to perform your normal routine. That is okay and there is no reason to feel guilty as long as you resume your activities without too long of a delay. Physical activity needs to be regular to produce benefits. You have worked hard to increase your physical fitness. The sooner you resume what you were doing the better you will feel.

Chapter 7

10 Common Sense Things to Do After a Fall

A fall by older person should never be thought of as a normal part of aging. Even if a fall does not result in serious injury, it can result in the "fear of falling." A "fear of falling" is characterized by feelings of dependency, loss of autonomy, loss of confidence in ambulation, and concern that future falls may have the potential for injury resulting in an additional loss of mobility.

Some patients avoid telling their doctor about a fall. One reason why patients avoid telling their doctor about a fall is they believe they'll be fast-tracked to an eventual loss of independence. The fact is, in those cases where patients are not forthcoming about a fall, they often place themselves at greater risk for future falls.

This chapter focuses on 10 pro-active steps to be taken after experiencing a fall. These steps help explore potential reasons for a fall and identify action that can be taken to lower future fall-risk.

Step 1. Meet with Your Doctor – Check for Any New Illnesses

Anyone who falls needs to be evaluated by a doctor. During the physical examination a doctor will be able to obtain a detailed history of the circumstance surrounding the fall. The physical exam will typically include; a gait assessment, sensory assessment (including hearing and vision) measurement of vital signs and neurological and musculoskeletal assessment. The exam may also include an evaluation of depression and cognitive impairment (1).

Step 2. Monitor Your Blood Pressure

Changes in blood pressure, such as postural hypotension, can lead to problems with gait and falls (2). Postural hypotension is defined as a decrease in systolic blood pressure of at least 20 mm Hg or a decrease in diastolic bold pressure of at least 10 mm Hg within 3 minutes of standing. If suggested by your doctor, monitoring blood pressure is an easy, non-invasive, inexpensive, and quick way to ensure changes in blood pressure do not place you at a risk for a fall.

Step 3. Understand Results of Completed Blood Tests

If your doctor performs blood tests, ask to review the results that are obtained. If there are any abnormal results from the blood tests, ask if the results could be related to an increased risk for falls.

For example, if you have diabetes and take insulin or other medications to lower blood sugar, an episode of low blood sugar (hypoglycemia) is an important risk factor for falls. Your doctor may suggest you closely monitor your blood sugar with a glucometer and maintain a blood sugar log.

Step 4. Conduct a Medication Review

Medication use by the older population has increased over the past few decades. It is estimated that 72% of people at least 55 years of age use at least one medication. In this age group, 20.3% are taking four or more medications (3). As a result, adverse drug reactions (ADR's) may occur and result in significant risk for falling.

It is important your doctor periodically review your list of medications to see if they are placing you at a risk for falls. If your medications are placing you at greater risk for falls, you may be offered recommendations on how best to take the medication to lower fall risk. If you are taking any the following medications ask for your doctor to review of how best to take these medications and lower fall risk:

1. **Sedatives, tranquilizers, or sleeping medications**.
   Examples of these medications include those for sleep and
   for anxiety. Antipsychotic medications for dementia
   behavior can increase sedation and elevate fall risk.

2. **Blood pressure and diabetes medications**.

3. **Opiate pain medications**

4. **Anticholinergic medications**. These include medications
   for allergies, overactive bladder, vertigo, nausea, and certain
   types of antidepressants which may be given for nerve pain.

Older adult drug prescriptions require on-going and close attention. This is especially important when there are multiple drug usage interactions that have the potential for increasing the risk for falls.

Step 5. Examine Gait and Balance

Gait and balance disorders are common in older adults and require a comprehensive assessment to determine contributing factors and appropriate interventions. Patients who report to their doctor that they have recently sustained a fall or are experiencing recurrent falls, present gait and balance abnormalities, or have difficulties with walking should undergo a comprehensive assessment (4), (5), (6), and (7).

Your doctor may recommend a physical therapist to conduct an evaluation and provide treatment suggestions for gait and balance disorders. A physical therapist will help in the identification of gait abnormalities and develop individualized plans to address functional issues presented (8), (9). Interventions that may be offered as part of physical therapy treatment include walking, functional exercise, and muscle strengthening techniques that have been determined to effective for improving balance (10).

Step 6. Dementia

It has been estimated by 2020, worldwide, there will be 42 million people with a diagnosis of dementia (11). Falls are a significant cause of injury in all older people but particularly those with dementia (12), (13). People with dementia recover more poorly after a fall than those without a diagnosis of dementia (14). Although dementia affects each person differently, people with dementia are at a greater risk for falls because they:

- Often have problems with mobility, balance and muscle weakness.
- Experience difficulties finding their way around.
- Have difficulties with processing events and situations.
- Are at greater risk for depression.
- Have increased difficulty expressing feelings, concerns, or needs.
- May be taking medications that make them drowsy or dizzy.

Communication is an important component for helping to reduce the risk of falls in those diagnosed with dementia. Some suggestions for communication with a person diagnosed with dementia include:

- Attempt to obtain eye contact with the person and reduce distractions.
- Watch closely for non-verbal cues that may help to identify intended actions and potential reactions.
- Use a calm and consistent approach. Use gentle gestures and pleasant facial expressions.
- Communicate instructions with short simple sentences.

- Consider the use of one-step-at-a-time activities. Allow sufficient time for the person to process information and, make frequent use of encouragement.

Step 7. Heart and Neurology

Falls in older people can be caused by underlying cardiovascular disorders (15). If you experience periods of blacking-out, losing consciousness or fainting you are at risk of having a fall that could result in serious injury. A loss of consciousness can be caused by an issue with the heart involving the rate the heart is beating or its rhythm. Problems with heart rate or rhythm may be caused by conditions such as:

Atrial fibrillation (an irregular heart rate)
Tachycardia (rapid heart rate)
Bradycardia (slow heart rate)

Many of these conditions can be successfully treated with medication and thereby lower your risk of injury. If you experience periods of a loss of consciousness, have blacked-out, fainted, or found yourself on the floor speak with you doctor about the symptoms you've experienced.

The nervous system consists of two components. The central nervous system consists of the brain and spinal cord. The peripheral nervous system is responsible for transmitting information between muscles, tissues, and the body to the brain. Impaired function of the peripheral nervous system may include symptoms such as numbness, tingling, and prickly sensations, sensitivity to touch or muscle weakness.

Neurological issues in older adults in the central and peripheral nervous system often present increased opportunities for falls. In one study it was determined that patients with stroke were six times more likely to suffer a fall than healthy patients in the control group. In the

74

same study, patients with Parkinson's disease were five times more likely to fall than those healthy patients in the control group. Others in the neurological fall risk categories that were four times higher risk for falls included those with dementia, epilepsy, other movement disorders, other vascular diseases, and peripheral neuropathy (16).

For those suffering from a central or peripheral nervous system disorder there should be an increased awareness of the potential for fall and injury. In many instances, to help lower the risk for a fall, physicians will recommend physical therapy for a gait analysis. The role of the physical therapist in the case of a neurological disorder is to identify opportunities to lower fall risk and enhance safe mobility.

Step 8. Vision Checks

It is well documented that visual function deteriorates with age and the loss of visual function increases fall risk (17). To help reduce some of the effects of aging, begin with having regular eye exams with an eye doctor such as an optometrist or ophthalmologist.

When meeting with your eye doctor discuss your medical history, the visual problems known to be in your family, and any visual problems you are experiencing. Your doctor should also be made aware of medications you are taking including non-prescription drugs, vitamins, herbals, and supplements.

Diabetes, high blood pressure, and cardiovascular disease increase the risk of age related eye diseases. The good news is that prevention is the best medicine for maintaining visual health and lowering fall risk. Prevention includes: regular exercise, non-smoking, avoiding intense ultraviolet light, monitoring sugar intake, good nutrition, and regular check-ups with your eye doctor.

Step 9. The Feet

With aging there are naturally changes to the feet. Similar to the rest of the body, muscle tissue in the feet tends to thin, blood begins to pool in veins, and the transmission of electrical impulses by nerves may change causing decreases in sensation. As a result, many falls experienced by older people result from age related deterioration of the balance and neuromuscular systems (18).

In an effort to help older people reduce fall risk it is important to encourage wearing well-fitting shoes both inside and outside the house. Older people who walk barefoot or in socks are at the greatest risk of falling (19).

Research recommendations indicate that older people should wear low-heel shoes, with a thin hard-sole to help maintain the best foot position. A softer sole is discouraged since it can make balance more difficult in challenging walking situations. Other recommendations include a tread sole and a treaded beveled heel that may lower fall risk on wet and slippery surfaces (19).

Step 10. Home Safety

In most instances, the location of a fall for an older person will be in the home (20). Therefore, it is important to determine if an element of the home environment may have been responsible for the fall.

Although a clean home is of the utmost importance, maintaining a clutter-free environment is an essential component for reducing fall risk. Chapter 8 of this book provides a home safety assessment checklist that identifies some common causes of falls. By utilizing a home safety assessment checklist, and making simple changes, it is possible to significantly improve home safety and lower fall risk.

Chapter Summary:

The desire to age in place necessitates the cause of a fall be investigated. For an older person even a minor fall can cause injury, result in hospitalization and potentially a lifetime of disability. Utilizing the 10 steps presented in this chapter will help in the identification of potential causes for a fall and steps to be taken to reduce future falls.

Chapter 8

Home Safety & Environmental Assessment

The *Home Safety and Environmental Assessment* tool was designed to assist caregivers and residents with the identification of the most common causes of falls. Although there are many potential medical issues that may cause a fall and injury, properly identifying and making environmental changes is a first step to improving senior home safety. The home assessments presented in this chapter identifies the five (5) most common areas in and around the home where falls occur.

#1 Home Entrances

Safe	Issue	N/A	Area Reviewed	Comments
✓	✓	✓		
			The primary doorway is visible (it is not obstructed by plants or shrubs).	
			Railings are securely mounted.	
			Outside lighting is present and working.	
			Primary door entrance has "peep-hole" for outside viewing.	
			Door locks in good working order (extra keys have been provided to essential caregivers).	
			Doorbell is working (determine if the bell can be heard from all areas of the home).	
			Walking surfaces are in good repair (free from cracks that present trip hazards). No broken steps or boards in need of replacement.	
			Outside areas where garbage is placed are free of trip hazards.	

- The importance of a clear line of site and pathway for entering and exiting the residence.

- Secure surfaces (railings) that allow the ability to safely ascend and descend steps and stairs.
- Security lighting that will allow the resident to see who is at the door
- Ability to see outside so as not to have to open the door to greet someone.
- Door locks that work properly and can be opened by those who visit the residence.
- A doorbell that can be heard from all areas of the residence.
- Outside surfaces that are frequently traveled (IE. to and from the mailbox) are free from trip hazards.
- Ability to remove trash from the residence without encountering potential safety hazards.

#1 Home Entrances (continued)

Safe	Issue	N/A	Area Reviewed	Comments
✓	✓	✓		
			If needed, the home is accessible by wheel chair and/or walker.	
			Outside walking surfaces are free of lubricants (oil, grease).	
			Essential pathways in the garage are unobstructed.	
			Garage lights are working and of proper intensity so as to permit night-time usage.	
			If present, the automatic garage door opener is in good working order.	
			Throw rugs are removed from garage floors.	
			Automatic sprinklers near doorways are in good working order (not flooding walking surfaces).	
			Yard surfaces where pets are taken are free of trip hazards (holes, hoses, sprinkler heads, etc).	

- The importance of wheel chair and walker accessibility to the residence. The resident should have the capability to access the residence without major difficulty.

- Surfaces should be free of chemical spills that may present slip hazards.
- The garage should permit easy access to the automobile and should be properly lighted so as to allow the resident to see at night and when the door is closed.
- Automatic garage doors should be checked to see if they are in proper working order and that the resident knows how to exit them if a power failure occurs.
- Loose rugs are removed from garage floor surfaces
- Automatic sprinklers can present safety hazards (in the winter months ice can form on paved surfaces).
- Yard areas are free of trip hazards (this is especially important for night-time walking of pets).

#2 Living Areas

Safe	Issue	N/A	Area Reviewed	Comments
✓	✓	✓		
			Doorways permit access for a wheel chair and/or walker.	
			Pathways are clear. If not, furniture can be re-arranged to permit the opening of a pathway.	
			No electric or phone cords are present in the open walking areas.	
			Light switches are easily accessible upon entry into the room (IE. without having to walk through a dark room).	
			Chair seating permits easy sitting and rising.	
			Primary seating is secure to the floor (no casters or wheels on furniture).	
			Telephone access is available in each room.	
			A working smoke detector is on each floor of the residence.	
			Windows are easy to open (IE. can be un-locked without difficulty).	
			Blinds and curtains are easy to open and close.	

- The resident should be able to move about the area without having to make special accommodation to enter or exit a room.

- Allow 42" or greater in all pathway areas in the home. Furniture that presents trip hazards should be moved out of common pathways.
- Extension, phone, or appliance cords should not be present in ambulation pathways.
- Entrances to rooms should provide lighting access.
- Chairs that require "low-seating" should be removed.
- Avoid the use of wheeled furniture (or furniture that is broken).
- Whenever possible, have phone availability in all rooms
- Ensure all smoke detectors are in proper working order.
- Windows should be easy to open and close.
- Blinds and curtains should easily allow the resident to open and close them so as to reduce glare.

#2 Living Areas (continued)

Safe ✓	Issue ✓	N/A ✓	Area Reviewed	Comments
			In rooms where glare is a problem can it be reduced (IE. install frosted bulbs, indirect lighting, shades on fixtures, or partially close blinds or curtains)?	
			Heating and air conditioning thermostats are easy to reach (and read).	
			All carpets are secured (no loose edges or throw-rugs).	
			Hallways are free of trip hazards (especially note clearance for walkers, canes, or a wheelchair).	
			Adequate lighting is present in all rooms (consider touring the home in the day-time and evening to inspect lighting).	
			Wood flooring is even with no trip hazards entering or exiting a room.	
			Terrazzo floors are clean and dry.	
			Pet food/water located in an area where they present no trip hazard.	
			Furniture (in high traffic areas) should be secure enough to be leaned-on.	

- All attempts should be made to reduce glare inside the residence. Glare negatively impacts visual capability in the elderly and increases the likelihood of a fall.
- A clear path to thermostats should be provided.
- Carpeting should be properly secured or removed
- All rooms should be adequately lighted.
- Flooring height differences should be noted and changes made if a trip hazard is present.
- Floors are clean and dry.
- Pet food, water, pet sleeping areas, and toys should not be walking obstacles.
- Any furniture that is used for stability (frequently grasped while ambulating through a room) should be secure to the floor. In particular check furniture that is on wood or terrazzo flooring. Also ensure chairs that are frequently used have secure arm rails.

#3 Bathrooms

Safe Issue N/A   Area Reviewed   **Comments**

✓	✓	✓		
			Will the doorway permit access by a walker* or wheelchair?**	
			Floor free of clutter (no throw rugs).	
			Toilet seat height appropriate for the primary resident (consider raising the seat if standing, sitting, or standing balance is a problem).	
			Grab bars installed in the shower, tub, and near the toilet.	
			Hot water temperature is safe (should be adjusted not to exceed 120 degrees Fahrenheit).	
			Shower bench seat is available.	
			Non-skid surface in the tub and shower.	
			Night light is present.	
			Towels, toilet paper, and personal supplies are easy to reach.	
			Hand-held shower wand available.	
			Examine opportunities to install a phone in the bathroom.	

*   If the bathroom will not permit forward entry with the use of a walker, it may allow side-ways entry.
** If the bathroom is not wheel chair accessible, a bedside commode may be an option.

In some residences walker and a wheelchair access into the bathroom is not possible. In other instances, however, turning the walker and ambulating "sideways" is possible. The important point to reinforce is that the resident must exercise great caution when forced to change ambulation direction to obtain entrance or exit the bathroom.

- Despite the dangers of water on the bathroom floor, all rugs must be secured to the floor.
- Toilet seat height must be appropriate to meet elder needs.
- Grab bars should be located in the shower, tub and near the toilet area.
- Water temperature should not present a burn hazard.
- Shower benches are very important for those with balance problems.
- Anti-"slip-strips" should be installed in the tub and shower.
- Nightlights should be installed in bathrooms.
- All "most frequently used" personal supplies should be easy to reach.
- Consider the installation of a hand-held shower wand.
- If opportunities are available, a phone in the bathroom is useful.

#4 Bedrooms

Safe	Issue	N/A	Area Reviewed	Comments
✓	✓	✓		
			Pathways clear throughout room.	
			Light switch is available at doorway entrance.	
			Light available on bedside stands (IE. should be one for each bed in room).	
			Floor free of clutter (no throw rugs).	
			Bed is firm and height adjusted to align with back of knees.	
			Chair in the room (with arm-rests).	
			Bedroom nightlight is installed.	
			Telephone access is near the bed.	
			Flash-light is close-by in the event of a power failure.	
			No rolling furniture is present.	
			Closet permits easy access to daily clothing items.	
			No electrical or phone cords are present as trip hazards.	

- As in other parts of the residence, attempt to have a 42" wide path clear of all trip hazards throughout the bedroom areas.
- Upon entering the room, the resident should be able to turn on a light without having to walk into a dark room.
- Rugs should be secured to the floor and all objects capable of creating a trip hazard should be removed from the floor.
- Bed height should allow for the resident to get easily in and out with minimal effort.
- Have at least one chair in the room with arm-rests.
- Install a nightlight near the bed that provides sufficient lighting of the floor surfaces.
- Provide a phone and flash-light on a bedside stand.
- Ensure all furniture is secured to the surface of the floor.
- Inspect the closet to ensure all essential clothing items are within reach
- Remove all electrical or phone cord trip hazards.

#5 Stairs

Safe	Issue	N/A	Area Reviewed	Comments
✓	✓	✓		
			Steps are clean and free of objects.	
			Every step properly fastened and clearly visible (IE. the edge of each step can be seen).	
			Steps are equal in height and depth.	
			Light switches are available at the top and bottom of the stairs. Lighting should not produce a glare.	
			Carpet is securely fastened. Avoid the use of deep-pile, dark colored, and patterned carpeting on stairs.	
			If there is no carpeting present, steps have non-skid strips in place.	
			A sturdy handrail is installed (handrails on both sides of the stairway is HIGHLY recommended especially if walking difficulties or other medical problems are present). Elders tend to rely more on rails as they descend stairs.	
			Shoes are worn going up and down stairs (IE. avoid wearing socks or smooth soled slippers or shoes.	

- Remove all objects from stairway surfaces
- Check for loose steps and ensure that each step is visible in all lighting situations.
- If steps are unequal in height, depth, or width, make sure the resident is aware of the differences.
- Light switches should be available at the top and bottom of the stairs. Check for sufficient lighting and for potential glare.
- Make sure all carpeting on stair surfaces is adequately secured. Install "skid-strips" in areas where the surface presents a slip hazard.
- Check the security of the rails. If possible, install a rail on both sides of the stairway.
- Encourage the use of shoes at all times when ascending or descending stairs.

#6 Kitchen

Safe	Issue	N/A	Area Reviewed	Comments
✓	✓	✓		
			Floor free of clutter (no throw rugs or mats)	
			Floor clean and dry and produces no glare (IE. no evidence of grease or other liquids on floor surface).	
			Appliances in good working condition (IE. all on/off indicator lights work).	
			Smoke detector working.	
			Storage spaces are easily accessible (IE. the most commonly used kitchen supplies are located between eye and knee levels).	
			All flammables are located away from heat sources.	
			Electrical outlets are not over-loaded.	
			Lighting sufficient for all kitchen activities.	
			Lighting switches are located at the primary entrance to the kitchen.	
			Appliances are un-plugged when not in use.	
			Drawers open and close without difficulty and are closed when not in use.	
			A step ladder (or step stool) is used to reach over-head objects in cabinets. Chairs should not be used for standing-on.	

- Floors should be clean and dry with no trip hazards. If a throw rug is near the sink, it should lie flat on the floor.
- Check stove and top burners to ensure on and off indicators are in good working condition.
- Inspect smoke detector to see that it is functioning properly
- Place the most frequently used kitchen utensils in a location that does not require significant over-head reaching.
- All flammables should be stored away from heat sources.
- Light switches are available upon entry into the kitchen
- Appliances are un-plugged when not in use.
- Drawers (including the dishwasher) are closed when not in use.
- A step ladder is used for reaching top cabinets. The use of a chair should be discouraged.

Your Home Survey Results

The goal for most of us is to remain living in our home as long as possible. The purpose of the review of your home is to identify six (6) areas where a potential hazard is present that could lead to a slip or trip and fall.

The following is the summary of the six (6) areas inside or outside your home where potential fall risks were identified:

Safety Topic	Potential Fall & Safety Issues
1. Home Entrances	_____
2. Living Area	_____
3. Bathrooms	_____
4. Bedrooms	_____
5. Stairs	_____
6. Kitchen	_____
Total	_____

Chapter Summary

The summary page is used to identify environmental areas and residential rooms that potentially may pose a safety problem. The Home Survey Results is designed to be a summary to call attention to areas where issues have been identified. The higher the number of problems in any area or room, the greater the safety risk.

A common misinterpretation of how to use this page is that a low number of identified issues indicates the area is safe. Remember, it only takes <u>one</u> "small issue" to cause a fall and injury. Risk is lessened only when all issues have been identified, corrective action has been taken, and risks are lessened to zero in each category.

Chapter 9

Life Part Two: An Example to Help Get You Started

Life Part Two outlines an approach to a healthier and happy retirement through identification of the essential areas and attitudes to focus upon. The book also highlights the importance of physical activity and personal safety with aging.

Having reviewed the information in the first 8 chapters you may be thinking it would be nice to have an example of how the information provided can be applied to your situation. The focus of this chapter is providing hypothetical healthcare issues that can be addressed utilizing the HAP model.

Retirement Example 1

Let's assume your health is good but you have a history of osteoarthritis in your family. In addition to this assumption, also assume your doctor believes your right knee is very arthritic and it is time to have the joint replaced.

A surgical joint replacement of your right knee is not something you'd really desire to do. However, it does have appeal because it will alleviate the pain you are experiencing while walking. The question is, "Can the HAP Model help you guide you through the transitional processes involved with the surgical procedure?"

To begin the answer this question let's start with a review of the model first discussed in Chapter 1. The 3 parts of the model are depicted as follows:

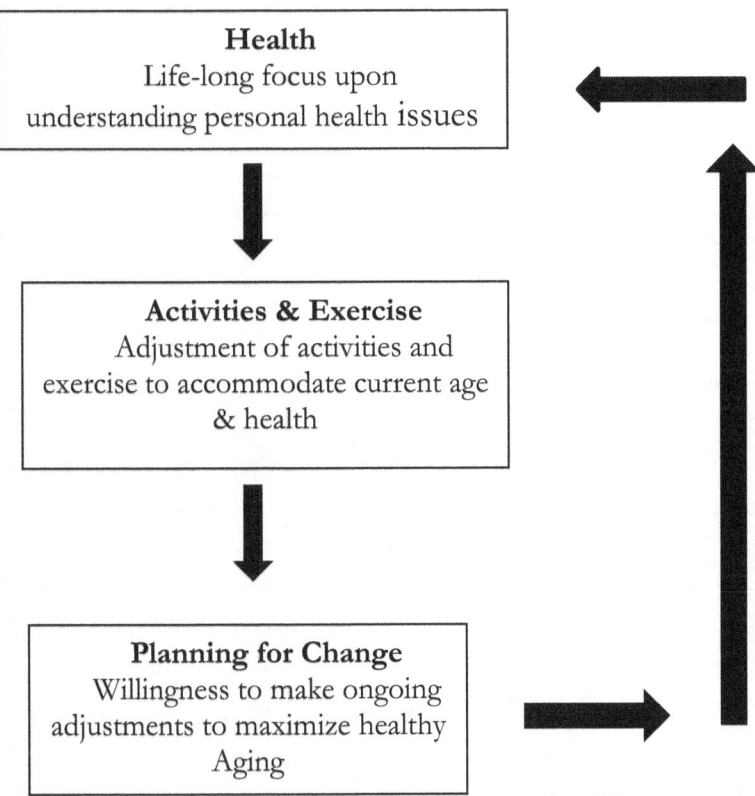

Beginning at the top of the model the first area to investigate is **Health.** In most instances, a total joint replacement surgery is performed on individuals greater than 60 years of age. To have a total joint procedure means you will be having the entire joint replaced in a single surgical procedure.

Utilizing the HAP model, your first step will be to investigate how osteoarthritis may affect your **Health** with aging. Your investigation may uncover osteoarthritis typically gets worse with ageing and leads to increased difficulty walking, climbing stairs, and often places you at greater risk of falls due to the on-going pain experienced.

Delaying the surgical procedure for an extended period may also adversely affect your health. If you decide not to have the procedure, worsening osteoarthritis may make it difficult to enjoy some of your current hobbies or limit your ability to visit and interact with your grandchildren.

Part of your pre-surgical investigation may include how the surgical procedure is performed, typical surgical risks, and rehabilitation outcomes. In other words, using the **Health** portion of the HAP model you will examine:

1. What osteoarthritis is and how it affects future health, mobility, and retirement.

2. How the surgical procedure is performed and what events typically transpire following the procedure.

Using the **Activities and Exercise** portion of the model you will investigate what expectations will be required of you following the procedure. For example, following the procedure, the primary focus of all healthcare **Activities** will be to ensure your get the maximum benefit from the new knee. The importance of obtaining the maximum benefit from the surgery is because the new joint is expected to last 10-20 years. Therefore, for the first few months following the surgery, it will be essential to perform the activities and exercises recommended by your physician and physical therapist.

In preparation for the procedure, your doctor may request you increase **Activity and Exercise** levels. Improving your physical health before an elective surgical procedure helps improve surgical recovery and outcome.

Planning for Change will involve preparation of your home environment. Your surgeon may suggest conducting a home safety assessment (Chapter 8) to make sure your home is ready and safe for your return. **Planning for Change** also includes ordering home safety equipment needed before returning home.

Planning for Change should include the development of short and long term goals (Chapter 3 and Appendix 1). Setting goals is a part of the transitional process and helps in the assessment of your current state of health and in making plans for how you want your health to evolve. Examples of short and long term goals for this surgical procedure might include the following:

Short Term Goal Examples

1. Return home as soon as possible from the hospital or rehabilitation facility with a good understanding of how to attain the best possible outcome.

2. Become independent in ambulation without the use of an assistive device such as a walker or cane in 2 months.

3. To be able to walk the dog outside in the front yard with no fear of falling in 2 months.

Long Term Goal Examples

1. To be able to play golf again in 3 months using an electric golf cart

2. In one year, to be able to return to walking safely on the uneven surfaces around the cabin in the woods and be able to take short hikes in the woods with the grandson.

Retirement Example 2

Health in this case involves a man that has over-all good health with the exception of longstanding low back pain. To resolve the

91

problem he underwent back surgery and, as a result, is feeling very well.

Activities and Exercise reflect he has always been very active performing yard work and repairs around his home. Regarding yard work, the surgeon who has been caring for his back has recommended he no longer engage in yard work. He currently has a very good outcome from the surgery and the surgeon is concerned that he may be no longer able to withstand the type of activities he does caring for his home without potentially damaging the surgical repair.

Planning for Change is difficult because he is presented with no longer having the capability to care for his home and yard he is being forced to step away from those responsibilities. He is also unable to afford paying the long term costs it will take to maintain the property.

Following the recommendations provided in Chapter 1, he decided to travel to other locations and see what types of accommodations were available. Once he located a new residence that required no outside maintenance on his part, he put his home up for sale and relocated to a comfortable retirement setting.

Retirement Example 3

Health involves a 78 year old female with a history of Type II diabetes with peripheral neuropathy in both lower extremities. Recently she has had increased difficulty with controlling her blood sugar levels despite taking medication and attempting to keep her weight down.

Activities and Exercise are walking approximately ½ mile per day outside of her home at a very relaxed pace with her dog and participating in Tai Chi twice a week to help maintain balance and flexibility. She met with her doctor who informed her that she must reduce her blood sugar level as quickly as possible or risk additional health problems commonly associated with diabetes.

Planning for Change was initiated following a discussion with her doctor. She indicated she would like to focus upon losing weight and begin a regular exercise program. She lives within 1 mile of a gym that is reasonably priced and has personal trainer services available.

In order to help her **Plan for Change**, the doctor recommended she meet with a personal trainer for several sessions to establish a well-rounded program that would safely accommodate her diabetic condition and lower extremity peripheral neuropathy. She began the program immediately and currently exercises three times a week for 45 minutes to an hour with each session. As a result of setting healthy short and long term goals she lost 10 pounds in the first two months and has made significant improvement in lowering and controlling her blood sugar levels.

Chapter Summary

The *HAP Model for Retirement Planning and Transition* is designed to encourage retirement self-examination and plan for future. The 3 components of the HAP model will remain constant throughout the aging process and always be in a state of transition. By utilizing the principles of the *HAP Model for Retirement Planning and Transition* it is anticipated the opportunity for having a healthier and happy retirement will greatly be increased.

Chapter 1 References

1. Kauppinen A: Meaning and happiness. Philosophical Topics 2013;41:161-185.

2. Mogilner C, Kamvar SD, Aaker J: The shifting meaning of happiness. Social Psychological and Personality Science, 2011;2(4): 395-402.

3. Mogilner C, Kamvar SD, Aaker J: The shifting meaning of happiness. Social Psychological and Personality Science, 2011;2(4): 395-402.

4. Drageset J, Haugan G, Treanag O: Crucial aspects promoting meaning and purpose in life: perceptions of nursing home residents. BMC geriatrics 2017; 17(1): 254.

5. Lynch, M., Wave, A. (2004) http://agewave.com/what-we-do/landmark-research-and-consulting/research-studies/new-retirement-survey/

6. Levy B, Slade M, Murphy T, Thomas M, Gill M: (2012). Association between positive age stereotypes and recovery from disability in older persons. JAMA 2012;308:(19): 1972-1973.

7. Epstein L, Steven M: The Harvard Medical School Guide to a Good Night's Sleep. McGraw-Hill, New York, 2007.

8. Klusmann V, Sproesser G, Wolff JK., Renner B: Positive self-perceptions of aging promote healthy eating behavior across the life span via social-cognitive processes. J Gerontol B Psychol Soc Sci, 2017;Nov 28.

9. Levy B, Slade M: Positive views of aging reduce risk of developing later-life obesity. Prev Med Rep, 2018:Dec 28;196-198.

10. Cohen, S: Social relationships and health. American Psychologist, 2004;59:676-684.

11. Kleiber D, Nimrod G: "I can't be very sad": Constraint and adaptation in the leisure of a "learning on retirement" group. Leisure Studies, 2009;28:67-83.

12. Kelly J. Leisure. Boston: Allyn & Bacon, 1996.

13. Coleman D, Iso-Ahola, SE: Leisure and health: The role of social support and self-determination. Journal of Leisure Research, 1993;25:111-128.

14. Carruthers CP, Hood CD: The power of the positive: Leisure and well-being. Therapeutic Recreation Journal, 2004;38: 225-245.

15. Pressman S, Mathews KA, Cohen S, Martire LM, Scheier M, Baum A, Schultz R: Association of enjoyable leisure activities with psychological and physical well-being. Psychosomatic Medicine, 2009;71:725-732.

16. Hutchinson SL, Nimrod G: (2012). Leisure as a resource for successful aging by older adults with chronic health conditions. The International Journal of Aging and Human Development, 2012; 74: 41-65.

17. Paillard-Borg S, Wang HX, Winblad B, Fratiglioni J: Pattern of participation in leisure activities among older people in relation to their health conditions and contextual factors: A survey in a Swedish urban area. Ageing and Society, 2009;29:803-821.

18. Silverstein M, Parker MG: Leisure activities and quality of life among the oldest in Sweden. Research on Aging, 2002;24:528-547.

19. Adams KB, Leibbrandt S, Moon H: A critical review of the literature on social and leisure activity and wellbeing in later life. Ageing & Society, 2011;31:638-712.

20. McConnell AR, Brown CM, Shoda TM, Stayton LE, Martin CE: Friends with benefits: on the positive consequences of pet ownership. J Pers Soc Psychol., 2001;Dec;101(6):1239-1252.

21. Powell L, Chia D, McGreevy P, Podberscek AL, Edwards KM, Neilly B, Guastella AJ, Lee V, Stamatakis E: Expectations for dog ownership: Perceived physical, mental and psychosocial health consequences among prospective adopters. PLoS One, 2018:Jul 6; 13(7).

22. Chowdhury EK, Nelson MR, Jennings GL, Wing LM, Reid CM: Pet ownership and survival in the elderly hypertensive population. J Hypertens, 2107;Apr;35(4):769-775.

23. Kelly J: Leisure. Boston: Allyn & Bacon, 1996.

24. Ogechi I, Snook K, Davis BM, Hansen AR, Lui F, Zhang J: (2016). Pet ownership and the risk of dying from cardiovascular disease among adults without major chronic medical conditions. High Blood Press Cardiovasc Prev, 2016;Sep23(3):245-253.

25. Ogechi I, Snook K, Davis BM, Hansen AR, Lui F, Zhang J: (2016). Pet ownership and the risk of dying from cardiovascular disease among adults without major chronic medical conditions. High Blood Press Cardiovasc Prev, 2016;Sep23(3):245-253.

26. Levy BR, Slade MD, Kunkel SR, Kasl SV: Longevity increased by positive self-perceptions of aging. Journal of Personality and Social Psychology, 2002;83(2):261-270.

Chapter 2 References

1. Cho AR, Moon JY, Kim S, An KY, Oh M, Jeon JY, Jung DH, Choi MH, Lee JW: Effects of alternate day fasting and exercise on cholesterol metabolism in overweight or obese adults: A pilot randomized controlled trial. Metabolism, 2019;Apr;93:52-60.

2. Med Sci Sports Exerc: American College of Sports Medicine position stand. Exercise and hypertension, 2004;Mar;36(3):533.

3. Pedersen BK.: Which type of exercise keeps you young? Curr Opin Nutr Metab Care, 2019;Mar;22(2):167-173.

4. Cadore EL, Pinto RS, Bottaro M, Izquierdo M. (2014). Strength and endurance training prescription in healthy and frail elderly. Aging Dis, 2014;Jun 1;5(3):183-195.

5. Parkkari J, Natri A, Kannus P, Manttari A, Laukkanen R, Haapasalo H, Pasanen M, Oja P, Vuori I: A controlled trial of the health benefits of regular walking on a golf course. Am J Med, 2000;Aug 1;109(2):102-108.

6. Palank EA, Hargreaves EH: The benefits of walking the golf course. Phys Sportsmed, 1990;Oct;18(10):77-80.

7. Middleton LE, Corbett D, Brooks D, Sage MD, Macintosh BJ, McIlroy WE, Black SE. Neurosci Biobehav Rev, 2013; Feb;37(2):133-137.

8. Mersy DJ: (1991). Health benefits of aerobic exercise. Postgrad Med, 1991;Jul;90(1):103-107,110-112.

9. Boutcher YN, Boutcher SH: Exercise intensity and hypertension: what's new? J Hum Hypertens, 2017; March3;31(3):157-164.

10. Morris M, Schoo A: Optimizing exercise and physical activity in older people. Butterworth Heinemann. NY. 2004;10.

11. Morris M, Schoo A: Optimizing exercise and physical activity in older people. Butterworth Heinemann. NY. 2004;10.

12. Brooks SV, Faulkner JA: Skeletal muscle weakness in old age: underlying mechanisms. Med Sci Sports Exerc, 1994April;26(4):432-439.

13. Kalish VB: Obesity in older adults. Prim Care, 2016, Mar;43(1):137-144.

14. Kligman EW, Pepin E: Prescribing physical activity for older adults. Geriatrics, 1992:Aug;47(8):33-34,37-44,47.

15. Macfarlane GJ, Lowenfels AB: Physical activity and colon cancer. Eur J Cancer, 1994:Sep;3(5):393-398.

16. Gilbert A, Czarkowska-Paczek B, Deptala A: (2013). Physical activity in prevention and treatment of colon cancer. Przegl lek, 2013:70(11):969-972.

17. Cong YJ, Gan Y, Sun HL, Deng J, Cao, SY, Xu X, Lu ZX: Association of sedentary behavior with colon and rectal cancer: a meta-analysis of observational studies. Br J Cancer, 2014; Feb4:110(3):817-826.

18. Brenner DR, Shaw E, Yannitsos DH, Warkentin MT, Brockton NT, McGregor SE, Town S, Hilsden RJ: Cancer Epidemiol, 2018;Apr;(53):12-20.

19. Gregg EW, Pereira MA, Caspersen CJ: Physical activity, falls, and fractures among older adults: a review of the epidemiologic evidence. J Am Geriatr Soc, 2000;Aug;48(8):883-893.

20. Menec VA, Chipperfield JG: Remaining active in later life; the role of locus of control in seniors' leisure activity participation, health and life satisfaction. J Aging Heal, 1997;9:105-125.

21. Mihalko SL, McAuley E: Strength training effects on subjective well being and physical function in the elderly. J Aging Physical Act 1996;4:56-68.

22. Rejeski WJ, Milhalko SL: Physical activity and quality of life in older adults. J Gerontology, 2001;56A:23-35.

Chapter 7 References

1. American Geriatrics Society (website) AGS/BGS clinical practice guidelines: prevention of falls in older persons (2010) New York, NY. American Geriatrics Society; 2011.

2. Mosnaim AD, Abiola R, Wolf ME, Perlmuter LC: Etiology and risk factors for developing orthostatic hypotension. Am J Ther 2010;17(1):86-91.

3. Ziere G, Dieleman J, Hofman Pols H, vander Cammen T, Stricker B: Polypharmacy and falls in middle age and elderly population. Br J Clin Pharmacol, 2006;61:218-223.

4. Rubenstein LZ, Powers CM, MacLean CH: Quality indicators for the management and prevention of falls and mobility problems in vulnerable elders. Ann Intern Med, 2001;135:686-693.

5. Ganz DA, Bao Y, Shekelle PG, Rubenstein LZ: Will my patient fall? JAMA, 2007;297(1):77-86.

6. American Geriatrics Society, British Geriatris Societ, and American Academy of Orthopaedic Surgeons Panel on Falls Prevention Guidline for the prevention of falls in older persons. J Am Geriatr Soc, 2001;49(5):664-672.

7. Chang JT, Ganz DA. Quality indicators for falls and mobility problems in vulnerable elders. J Am Geriatr Soc, 2007;55(sup 2):5327-5334.

8. Harris MH, Holden MK, Cahalin LP, Fitzpatrick D, Lowe S, Canavan PK: Gait in older adults: a review of the literature with an emphasis toward achieving favorable outcomes. part I. Clin Geriatrics, 2008;16(7):33-42.

9. Harris MH, Holden MK, Cahalin LP, Fitzpatrick D, Lowe S, Canavan PK: Gait in older adults: a review of the literature with an emphasis toward achieving favorable outcomes. part II. Clin Geriatrics, 2008; 16(8):37-45.

10. Howe TE, Rochester L, Jackson A, Banks PM, Blair VA: (2007). Exercise for improving balance in older people. Cochrane Database Syst Rev, 2007;(4):CD004963.

11. Ferri CP, Prince M, Brayne C, Brodaty H, Fratiglioni l, et al. Global prevalence of dementia: a Delphi consensus study. Lancet, 2005;366:2112-2117.

12. Morris JV, Rubin EH, Morris EJ, Mandel SA: Senile dementia of the Alzheimer's type: an important risk factor for serious falls. Journal of Gerontology, 1987;42:412-417.

13. van Doorn C, Gruber-Baldini AL, Zimmerman S, Herbel JR, Port CL, et al: Dementia as a risk factor for falls and fall injuries among nursing home residents. Journal of the American Geriatrics Society, 2003;51:1213-1218.

14. Shaw FE: Falls in cognitive impairment and dementia. Clinics in Geriatric Medicine, 2002;18:159-173.

15. Tan MP, Kenny RA. Cardiovascular assessment of falls in older people. Clin Interv Aging, 2006; Mar;1(1):57-66.

16. Homann B, Plaschg A, Grundner M, Haubenhofer A, Griedl T, Ivanic G, Hofer E, Fazekas F, Homann N: The impact of neurological disorders on the risk for falls in the community dwelling elderly: a case-controlled study. BMJ Open, 2013;3(11):e003367. Published online.

17. Saftari LN, Kwon OS: Ageing vision and falls: a review. J Physiol Anthropol, 2018;37:11. Published online 2018 Apr 23.

18. Lord SR, Sherrington C, Menz HB: Falls in older people: Risk factors and strategies for prevention. 2nd ed. Cambridge (England): Cambridge University Press, 2001.

19. Menant JC, Steele JR, Menz HB, Munro BJ, Lord SR: Optimizing footwear for older people at risk of falls. J Rehabilitation Research & Development, 2008;45;Nov8;1167-1182.

20. Pfortmuller CA, Kunz M, Linder G, Zisakis A, Puig S, Exadaktylos AK: Fall related emergency department admission: fall environment and settings and related injury patterns in 6357 patients with special emphasis on the elderly. ScientificWorldJournal, 2014;Mar 2:256519.

Appendix 1 – Goal Setting

Short Term Goals:

1._____

_____

_____

_____

2._____

_____

_____

_____

Long Term Goals:

1._____

_____

_____

_____

2._____

_____

_____

_____

Appendix 2 – Endurance Activity Record

Week of:	Activity	Length of Time
Monday		
Tuesday		
Wednesday		
Thursday		
Friday		
Saturday		
Sunday		

Notes:_____

_____

_____

_____

Appendix 3 – Exercise Tracking Chart

Week of:	Exercise 1:	Exercise 2:	Exercise 3:	Exercise 4:	Exercise 5:
Monday					
Tuesday					
Wednesday					
Thursday					
Friday					
Saturday					
Sunday					

Index

About the Author

Mark A. Brimer Ph.D. is a heath care risk manager and physical therapist who has been involved in healthcare for nearly 40 years. He is a multi-book author and co-author and has served as an expert witness in medical malpractice cases throughout the United States.

Mark has volunteered for the Florida Department of Health and the Florida Department of Elder Affairs in the identification of opportunities to reduce senior injuries. As two term Mayor of the City of Satellite Beach, Florida, he placed great emphasis on local government identification of opportunities to enhance the capability for aging citizens to remain in their residence for as long as possible.

As a result of his on-going community services efforts for seniors, Mark was recognized as a *Jefferson Award recipient for Outstanding Public Service*. As of this writing, Mark remains active in the identification and implementation of opportunities to enhance "Aging in Place" and home safety for seniors.

www.ingramcontent.com/pod-product-compliance
Lightning Source LLC
Chambersburg PA
CBHW051445280526
45785CB00003B/1428